Managing healthcare — law and practice

Butterworths **Tolley**
LexisNexis™

Members of the LexisNexis Group worldwide

United Kingdom	LexisNexis Butterworths Tolley, a Division of Reed Elsevier (UK) Ltd, 2 Addiscombe Road, CROYDON CR9 5AF
Argentina	LexisNexis Argentina, BUENOS AIRES
Australia	LexisNexis Butterworths, CHATSWOOD, New South Wales
Austria	LexisNexis Verlag ARD Orac GmbH & Co KG, VIENNA
Canada	LexisNexis Butterworths, MARKHAM, Ontario
Chile	LexisNexis Chile Ltda, SANTIAGO DE CHILE
Czech Republic	Nakladatelství Orac sro, PRAGUE
France	Editions du Juris-Classeur SA, PARIS
Hong Kong	LexisNexis Butterworths, HONG KONG
Hungary	HVG-Orac, BUDAPEST
India	LexisNexis Butterworths, NEW DELHI
Ireland	Butterworths (Ireland) Ltd, DUBLIN
Italy	Giuffrè Editore, MILAN
Malaysia	Malayan Law Journal Sdn Bhd, KUALA LUMPUR
New Zealand	Butterworths of New Zealand, WELLINGTON
Poland	Wydawnictwo Prawnicze LexisNexis, WARSAW
Singapore	LexisNexis Butterworths, SINGAPORE
South Africa	Butterworths SA, DURBAN
Switzerland	Stämpfli Verlag AG, BERNE
USA	LexisNexis, DAYTON, Ohio

© Reed Elsevier (UK) Ltd 2002

A CIP Catalogue record for this book is available from the British Library.

ISBN 0 406 947031

Typeset by Columns Design Ltd, Reading, England
Printed and bound in Great Britain by Hobbs the Printers

Visit Butterworths LexisNexis *direct* at www.butterworths.com

Key references

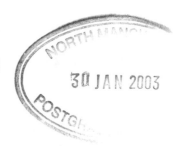

The following references are essential background for readers of this handbook. All can be downloaded free of charge from the website addresses given.

Department of Health (1997) *The New NHS: Modern, Dependable,* HMSO, London (*www.doh.gov.uk/nnhsind.htm*)

Department of Health (1998) *A First Class Service: Quality in the new NHS,* HMSO, London (*www.doh.gov.uk/nnhsind.htm*)

Department of Health (2000) *The NHS Plan: A plan for investment, a plan for reform,* HMSO, London (*www.doh.gov.uk/nhsplan*)

Department of Health (2000) *An Organisation with a Memory,* HMSO, London (*www.doh.gov.uk/orgmemreport*)

Department of Health (2001) *Building a Safer NHS for Patients,* HMSO, London (*www.doh.gov.uk/buildsafenhs)*

Department of Health (2001) *Doing Less Harm – Improving the safety and quality of care through reporting, analysing and learning from adverse incidents involving NHS patients* Version 1.0a, draft document (*www.npsa.org.uk)*

Department of Health (2001) *Learning from Bristol: the report of the public inquiry into children's heart surgery at the Bristol Royal Infirmary 1984–1995,* Command Paper CM 5207, HMSO, London (*www.bristol-inquiry.org.uk*)

NHS Executive (1999) *Guidelines for Implementing Controls Assurance in the NHS,* NHSE, Leeds, November 1999 (*www.doh.gov. uk/riskman.htm).* The controls assurance website also features the latest controls assurance standards.

Turnbull N and working party (1999) *Internal Control – Guidance for Directors on the Combined Code (The Turnbull Report),* Institute of Chartered Accountants in England and Wales, London (*www.icaew.co.uk/internalcontrol*)

Foreword

For the first forty years or so in the existence of the National Health Service, the quality of the services provided was not a widely debated subject outside those with an academic or specialist interest. Quality was an implicit rather than explicit part of day-to-day service delivery, as it now is for both the NHS and the private healthcare sector. Management attention was focused on achieving higher activity levels and using resources more efficiently.

In the late 1990s the concept of clinical governance was born – establishing as a fundamental principle that all NHS organisations should have in place proper systems to assure and improve the quality of services they provided. Clinical governance is underpinned by a statutory duty of quality enshrined in an Act of Parliament. Implementing a programme of clinical governance requires a big shift for a hospital or a primary care service: a transformation in culture, in operating systems and working practices together with a refocusing of all activity to the needs and experience of the patient.

A key strand of clinical governance is patient safety, another concept which healthcare systems around the world have come to recognise relatively late. An emphasis on patient safety also requires a change in organisational culture – to one which emphasises an approach based upon learning from error rather than blame and punishment, which encourages reporting and which provides a strong bedrock of information on adverse events and near-misses.

At the core of the drive to improve patient safety is promoting a greater understanding of risk in healthcare and the management of risk. This is no longer the domain of specialist 'risk managers'. It is everybody's business. Without a full appreciation of the vulnerability in the systems of an organisation it cannot be made a safer place for patients.

This book is an excellent review of this important field, offering readers new to the subject as well as existing specialists a clear and comprehensive guide to the assessment and management of risk in healthcare.

Sir Liam Donaldson
Chief Medical Officer
Department of Health

Contents

Contents

Contents

Contents

About the Authors

General editor:

Dr Vanessa L Mayatt, BSc PhD DipOHS FRSH MIOSH RSP

Vanessa is an independent risk management consultant and board member of the Public Health Laboratory Service. Previous posts held include health and safety director for PPP Healthcare and AXA Assistance, healthcare practice leader for Marsh, health and safety practice leader for Marsh, visiting fellow at Salford University's European Occupational Health and Safety Law Research Centre and NHS trust unit director for Sedgwick. Prior to joining Sedgwick, she was HM principal specialist inspector of health and safety within HSE. Vanessa has worked with the healthcare sector in her various roles since 1984 and has extensive experience of helping the sector to manage risk. She has lectured widely in this country and abroad on risk management, including the management of occupational health and safety and clinical risk. She has many publications to her name. Vanessa has been a member of the *Health Care Risk Report* editorial board since 1995.

Chapter authors:

Mary Burrows, BSc MBA MBE

Mary is chief executive of Northampton Primary Care Trust, which commissions and provides services for the local population. She is an American citizen but has spent the last 12 years in the UK. During this time she has worked mainly in acute hospital care, spending nine years at the Oxford Radcliffe Hospitals NHS Trust in senior management positions before moving into primary care in 2000. Mary has over 20 years experience of clinical practice and management in the UK and US. She has been a member of the Health and Safety Commission's Health Services Advisory Committee and, in 1996, was awarded a MBE in recognition of her risk management achievements in the NHS.

Jo Wilson, MSc PGDip BSc FCIPD MHSM AIRM RGN RM RSCN ENB 400

Jo is European healthcare director for Marsh. Jo has worked as a clinical risk and quality management consultant for Marsh and previously HRRI and its forerunner company HRS, for over 10 years. She has held several posts within the NHS, the most recent being regional resource management nurse and quality facilitator for the Northern Region. Her NHS and consultancy posts have given her wide experience of clinical practice, quality improvements and risk management within the healthcare sector, both in the UK and internationally. Jo has published and lectured extensively and is a lecturer/practitioner at Nottingham Law School, Nottingham Trent University. She is a member of the editorial boards for *Health Care Risk Report* and the *British Journal of Nursing* and an external reviewer for the *Nursing Times, NT Research* and the *British Journal of Nursing*.

Trevor Payne, MSc BIFM MHEFMA

Trevor is head of facilities at the Oxford Radcliffe Hospitals NHS Trust, one of the largest acute teaching hospitals in the UK. He has a professional engineering background having trained in both Electrical and Plant Engineering and subsequently gaining a MSc in Facilities Management at Strathclyde Graduate Business School. Trevor is a seasoned lecturer and presenter of papers in international fora. He has also written and contributed to a number of books in his field. He is a member of the editorial board of *Facilities Management*.

Graham E Offord, MCBIS MBCI AIRM

Graham has worked in the risk management arena for 15 years. For the last 10 years he has focused as a consultant on business continuity. Graham currently works within the Business Continuity Management Consultancy Team in Marsh. Over the years he has been instrumental in the implementation of business continuity plans across various work sectors throughout Europe, including the UK. Graham's particular areas of expertise include business continuity policy, strategy and implementation, risk analysis and business impact and risk management measures to protect organisations.

Janet Martin, BA FCIPD

Janet works as an employment specialist providing helpline advice and guidance to NHS and independent healthcare employers on employment and human resource issues. She also works within the Eastern Deanery as a human resource consultant which involves her in the appointment of doctors in training, assessment and appeal arrangements and the provision of training in equality and interview skills. Janet has worked in the NHS in a number of human resource roles dealing with employment relations and organisational change issues.

1 General introduction

Dr Vanessa L Mayatt

Risk management is central to the effective running of any organisation. Within the healthcare sector, risk management has never been more topical. The recent incidents associated with healthcare delivery, where risk has been poorly managed and patients harmed, are almost too many to mention. The intense media coverage of these incidents has repeatedly drawn public attention to failures in healthcare delivery, whether isolated incidents involving one patient, or poor practice over time involving many patients. Whilst newspapers are sold on the strength of these stories, no one else wins, especially not patients, healthcare organisations or the individuals working within them. This alone should be a strong motivator for effective risk management.

Why is managing risk important?

All organisations are currently required to operate against the backdrop of many externally driven requirements to manage risk. These include corporate governance, insurance-related risk management programmes and legal duties. For healthcare organisations, controls assurance, clinical governance, CNST, NICE, CHI, MDA and HSE initiatives need all to be added. These many external pressures require the implementation of best practice in managing healthcare organisations and their attendant risks.

External pressures apart, there are other good reasons for managing risk and there are dividends to be reaped from doing so. Increasingly, healthcare organisations are seeing the benefit of managing risk in the quality of patient care, in staff/patient relationships, in staff morale and also financially. Whilst the nature of the external pressures ensures that managing risk is not optional, a genuine organisation-wide belief that risk management is central to looking after patients, staff and ensuring business survival is the best motivator.

Keeping abreast of changes

Managing risk in healthcare is a fast-moving field. The precise nature and specific requirements of the various external drivers are subject to continual change and development. The pace of these changes is swift. Risk management is an iterative process necessitating constant endeavour to secure ever better standards. Staff working in healthcare organisations as risk management professionals or with responsibility for managing risk, therefore, have a sizeable task to keep abreast of developments on all fronts, to understand what has to be done and then to secure effective implementation.

Aims of this book

This publication originated from a desire to provide a comprehensive and up-to-date steer through the key legal and best practice requirements relevant to managing risk in the healthcare sector. The overall aim of the handbook is therefore to provide up-to-date guidance on managing specific areas of risk. The handbook has been written from a practical standpoint by individuals who are both expert in managing risk and have extensive experience of the successful implementation of risk management initiatives in healthcare organisations. All the contributors have set out to demystify the complexities and challenges that are encountered when embarking upon or further developing risk management initiatives. There is much reinvention of the wheel in devising risk management initiatives in the healthcare sector. This handbook aspires to set out the expert views of the various contributors so that experience is shared and healthcare organisations can more efficiently enhance the means by which they manage risk in practice.

Structure of the book

Key references and guidance

Current key documents and guidance, such as Department of Health reports, as well as essential references are set out on page iii. At the end of each chapter, other main reference sources are listed. A glossary of the main terms used throughout the chapters is on p227.

Managing risk

The guidance commences at chapter 2. This chapter, written by Mary Burrows, contains general guidance on managing risk. For those new to this field, this is an important chapter to start with. For those more experienced in risk management, this chapter should still prove interesting and useful, as it contains many practical pointers to achieving best practice. The chapter explains the relationship between risk management and the related initiatives of clinical and corporate governance, controls assurance and quality. This is done in order to encourage a combined approach to these various initiatives rather than dealing with each separately.

Incident reporting

One of the most important aspects of managing risk is the recording of incidents, their analysis to check performance and identify priorities and then investigation to learn lessons and implement change. In recognition of the importance of this aspect of managing risk, this topic is addressed next in chapter 3. In this chapter, Mary Burrows covers an area with which many healthcare organisations struggle and, consequently, waste much time and energy on. The chapter straddles all areas of risk and will therefore have wide appeal to individuals with risk management responsibilities as well as those with a general interest. The chapter is practically based and contains many excellent tips for the successful implementation of incident recording systems.

The so-called blame culture, whilst not unique to healthcare, has undoubtedly played its part in reducing levels of reported incidents, the factual accuracy of reports and the ability to learn lessons. Chapter 3 explains the importance of establishing a blame-free culture and how this can be achieved in practice.

Clinical risk and clinical governance

Chapter 4 from Jo Wilson deals specifically with the management of clinical risk. The related area of clinical governance is covered by the same author in chapter 5. The aim of chapter 4 is to enhance understanding of how clinical risk can arise, and therefore be prevented, and the organisational and human factors that impinge upon clinical risk and its consequences.

Incidents of clinical negligence typically attract significant media attention and are often associated with claims for compensation. The number of claims has steadily increased over the last decade as indeed have the value of settlements, particularly, but not exclusively, in obstetric cases. Failing to manage clinical risk does therefore cost the healthcare sector dearly, both in financial terms and in terms of the impact on individuals – both patients and their families, and clinicians, their families and colleagues. Chapter 4 addresses the causes of negligence claims and how they may be avoided. It also contains practical advice on best practice in relation to claims management.

NHS trusts in England have been members of the Clinical Negligence Scheme for Trusts (CNST) since its inception in the early 1990s. This is a major initiative in the clinical risk management arena. Awareness of the CNST's risk management standards both for CNST members and organisations outside of England is clearly important in developing approaches to managing clinical risk. Chapter 4 therefore provides some background in relation to the CNST and the latest developments with its risk management standards. The chapter goes on to deal with effecting change in practice following clinical incidents.

Chapter 5 concentrates on the principles and key elements of clinical governance, the current requirements and their relationship to clinical risk management and controls assurance. The chapter also addresses the roles of relevant bodies such as the National Institute for Clinical Excellence (NICE) and the Commission for Health Improvement (CHI).

Managing health, safety and environmental risks

In chapter 6, I deal with the management of health, safety and environmental risks. This chapter covers the diverse nature of these risks in healthcare organisations and the consequences of failing to manage them effectively. The principles of effective management and how to establish management systems are also explored. Legislation and good practice guidance in this field is under constant development. The requirements of the main pieces of current legislation are addressed, together with how to comply with these legal requirements. There are several major initiatives in the health, safety and environmental arena that are currently vital to incorporate into any strategy to tackle these areas of risk. These major initiatives are covered together with the anticipated changes in corporate manslaughter legislation. In many healthcare organisations, health, safety and environmental risks are separated from measures to address other areas of risk, in particular clinical risk. Arguments are put forward for merging approaches to these two areas and some of the consequences of failing to do so are highlighted.

Managing the physical environment

The challenges to managing the physical environment and the detail of good management in this area are the focus of Trevor Payne in chapter 7. Healthcare is delivered from a diverse range of settings in terms of size, complexity, age, design and maintenance standards. The nature and quality of the healthcare environment can have a direct bearing on the wellbeing of staff and patients. Indeed, if the physical environment is not up to standard, lives can be placed at risk, as has happened in the past. Estates and facilities management is a specialised field, subject to rapid change and is therefore no different from other areas of risk associated with healthcare delivery. Outsourcing, insourcing, PFI-funded developments and Public/Private Partnerships (PPP) are all part of the current territory of specialists in this field. Managing contractors and consortium relationships are challenges for any organisation, but are nonetheless crucial to get right so that money is not wasted, project deadlines are achieved and high quality patient care delivery is assured.

Service continuity management

Over recent years, the healthcare sector has experienced a number of major incidents. These have included multiple deaths from an outbreak of Legionnaires' disease, hospital-acquired infection affecting both patients and staff, and collapse of patient administration systems. Whilst these major incidents are not daily occurrences, they do unfortunately reoccur and on each occasion have a major impact upon service delivery. In chapter 8, Graham Offord tackles service continuity planning, the impact of disasters within healthcare and resourcing for disaster recovery. Successful service continuity management requires input from individuals with differing backgrounds and skills. This chapter contains good practice advice that will appeal to a diverse range of roles in the healthcare sector.

Managing people

The final chapter deals with managing people. People are any organisation's most important asset and this is never more true than within healthcare. Janet Martin covers some of the recent high profile incidents with healthcare and the resultant changes to personnel management practice. Her chapter illustrates the wide-ranging impact upon the delivery of healthcare if staff recruitment, training, CPD programmes, resourcing and skill mix are not right. She explains how to establish and implement good standards in managing people.

Future editions of this book

Any publication that claims to cover the latest initiatives and current developments, will naturally be out of date, at least in some respects, the moment it is published. This is especially so for the subject matter of this publication as the entire arena of managing risk in healthcare is constantly changing. For the future it is planned that the publication will be regularly updated and the guidance within the individual chapters expanded, so that healthcare organisations have continued access to up-to-the-minute, practical and quality advice.

2 Managing risk

Mary Burrows

This chapter covers:

- **The concept of risk management**
- **Eight principles of risk management**
- **Assessing risk, taking action and performance monitoring**
- **Risk, quality and controls assurance**
- **Risk strategy**
- **Consequences of not managing risk**

Risk management as a concept was introduced into the NHS in the 1990s as a means of identifying and addressing risks that are present in the provision of healthcare. Many readers may think that it is a rather dull subject and, depending on how it is approached and discussed, it can be. However, risk management does present a positive opportunity to bring about change within an organisation and to allow professionals to challenge the way they think and behave.

Early risk management guidance targeted at the healthcare sector tended to focus on estates, facilities, health, safety and disaster management. For many healthcare professionals, it seemed to bear little relevance to the treatment and diagnosis of patients. Many of those same professionals lost sight of the fact that hospitals and even general practice are industries in their own right with a multitude of risk management issues to address – not just clinical ones. It is now generally recognised that risk management applies to all areas of risk associated with healthcare provision, including clinical practice.

This chapter addresses the following issues:

- definitions and principles of risk management
- how risk arises in healthcare
- the relationship of risk with governance and quality

- how risk management can be applied within the healthcare setting

The aim is to give readers the ability to:

- define and understand the principles of risk management

- identify, assess and control risks

- understand how risk management fits with governance, controls assurance and quality

- develop and introduce risk management into their organisation

- understand and accept the consequences of not managing risk

The history of risk

Risk, as a concept, can be traced back over many centuries. It first manifested itself in gambling, but through the application of many of the great minds throughout the last five centuries, it became more fully understood.

References to uncertainty and risk can be found in ancient Greek literature and mythology, but the Greeks did not develop it as a theory. Instead they relied on what was factual and proven, looking to the Gods for outcomes. In other words, they relied on luck and instinct for how decisions were made.

Risk today

Our concept of risk can be found in the Indo-Arabic numbering system of some 800 years ago. The foundation of risk is thus based on mathematical probability. But it is in the Renaissance period that we find the emergence of risk as a more serious subject concerned with forecasting the future through informed decision-making. Whilst we may consider that we apply some of the Greeks' reliance on luck and instinct today in our own lives, the truth is we make informed decisions. We make choices about how to behave because the probabilities of various outcomes have already been determined and are in the public domain. A good illustration of this is the use of seatbelts and the risk of death in a road traffic accident if not worn. Whilst few of us may be able to quote any statistics, it is engendered in our society to the extent that very few people will take the risk and instead will wear their seatbelts when driving. The law has solidified this societal view by making it unlawful to drive without seatbelts.

It is the origin of the word 'risk' itself that perhaps explains the essence and importance of it. Risk is derived from the early Italian word *risicare* which means 'to dare'. Risk therefore takes on a sense of individual responsibility alluding to a choice that a person makes rather than a reliance on fate, superstition or instinct.

The science and subjectivity of risk

At the beginning of the 20th century a scientific approach was applied to understanding risk. During this time the substantive link between risk and uncertainty was identified, first by Willett[1] and later by Knight.[2] It is the work of the latter that provides our basis for a classical approach to risk based on management science theory. Knight observed that a person had three key advantages in decision-making if management science theory was applied. These were:

- knowledge of the problem itself

- an understanding of the complete range of possible outcomes

- the ability to objectively assess the likelihood of each outcome occurring.

But Knight only went so far in his theory because he excluded unmeasurable uncertainty – the truly unforeseen. A good example of the importance of the unforeseen, especially in 20th century medicine, is the devastating damage to children as a result of thalidomide use during pregnancy.

Knight also assumed that assessment of any likelihood (probability) is objective, when in fact it can be subjective. We must therefore accept that whilst risk and the management of risk is a science, it is not a perfect one in the sense that it is difficult, if not impossible, to separate risk from uncertainty. Risk management is therefore an imprecise science.

In work researched and produced by Bettis,[3] risk and the diversity of risk in organisations was studied. The conclusion was that if risk is applied to financial theory, it could easily be described by using a number of methods, the probabilistic distribution of market returns as one example. It is a mathematical solution and follows a precise, well-defined theory. However, when risk is applied to an organisation and decision-making within it, it pertains more to how a manager applies judgment and the consequences of their decisions. So, for the first time, human factors such as behaviour enter the discussion. Once subjectivity arises, uncertainty is inevitable.

Defining risk

Does a definition of risk really matter given the associated confusion and complexity? Are precise definitions necessary or is it general concepts we should be more concerned about?

The distraction that often crops up, even in healthcare, is the emphasis on trying to define risk and the extent of it in such a precise way that it becomes the end as opposed to a means to an end. That is not to say that determining probabilities is not important – indeed, parts of health and safety legislation require that this is done – but it is only one part of risk management. This is a subject revisited later in this chapter, in the discussion of the development and implementation of a risk management strategy.

It is the understanding of risk and uncertainty that is crucial to addressing risk in healthcare, whether applied to the organisation, the environment or the people involved or affected. A simple working definition of risk is:

"the probability or likelihood that harm may occur, coupled with the consequences of that harm"

Such harm could manifest itself in a number of ways, such as social exclusion, physical or psychological damage or financial impact. These concepts are discussed further in the sections that follow.

Principles of risk management

This section addresses the principles of risk management, and then provides a step-by-step guide to risk management. This structured approach will enable subsequent chapters to be set in context, with a background of essential skills in place.

At its simplest, risk management is good management practice. It should not be seen as an end in itself, but as part of an overall management approach applicable to any organisation. There are eight guiding principles concerning risk:

> **Principles of risk management**
>
> 1. A culture where risk management is considered an essential and positive element in the provision of healthcare.
> 2. Risk reduction and quality improvement should be seen as activities worthy of being pursued.
> 3. Risk management often works within a statutory framework which cannot be ignored.
> 4. A risk management approach should provide a supportive structure for those involved in adverse incidents or errors by enabling a no-blame culture.
> 5. Processes should be strengthened and developed to allow for better identification of risk.
> 6. Managing risk is both a collective and an individual responsibility.
> 7. Recognise that resources may sometimes be required to address risk.
> 8. Every organisation should strive to understand the causes of risk, its link with quality and the importance of addressing issues.

Principle 1 – a culture where risk management is considered an essential and positive element in the provision of healthcare

Risk spans all functions in an organisation. However, since risk management is still seen to be in development when applied to clinical care and practice, many healthcare professionals may still think it relates to estate or health and safety issues (hereafter referred to as non-clinical risk).

Fortunately this perception is rapidly changing, with healthcare professionals more aware of the concept of risk and the importance that managing risk plays in the development and delivery of care. It is therefore important that rather than adopting two risk management approaches, one for clinical risk and another for non-clinical, one integrated approach should be adopted. This will ensure that important concerns do not get buried simply because a decision could not be made as to whether the risk was clinical or non-clinical.

Principle 2 – risk reduction and quality improvement should be seen as activities worthy of being pursued

Many healthcare organisations are already subject to review through the application of high-level performance indicators (HLPIs), visits by Royal

11

Colleges, and inspections by the Health and Safety Executive (HSE). Some have already come under review by the Commission for Health Improvement (CHI) and others will do so over a four-year timescale.

With the creation of the National Institute of Clinical Excellence (NICE), the CHI, national service frameworks (NSFs) and the NHS Executive controls assurance requirements, demonstration of how standards are met in healthcare delivery is becoming increasingly important as a performance measure. By applying the risk management approach as a route to improving quality, complying with the various standards will become much easier than perhaps originally envisaged.

Principle 3 – risk management often works within a statutory framework that cannot be ignored

A statutory framework is not confined to health and safety, but embraces all aspects of the healthcare function from employment law through to the *Health Act 1999* and its statutory duties for quality and working in partnership. The introduction of the *Human Rights Act 1998* illustrates the need for employers and employees to be aware of their legal obligations. By adopting a risk management approach, statutory obligations can be identified and fulfilled in a positive way, rather than as a means of avoiding litigation and prosecution.

A strategy should account for the extent to which education and development of staff is necessary so that they understand what is required of them, and thus take responsibility for working within the law in its widest sense.

Principle 4 – a risk management approach should provide a supportive structure for those involved in adverse incidents or errors by enabling a no-blame culture

For too many years the NHS and other public bodies have operated a culture of blame; this is evident in the language used and the way issues are approached when things have gone wrong. Many in the public sector have worked consistently over the years, and with some success, to overcome this negative culture by objectively looking at why an error or adverse event occurred, supporting staff and patients through the process and seeking improvements where possible.

A good risk management approach looks beyond the negatives and is open, overcomes the problems of professional boundaries and focuses on improving safety for all rather than seeking and allocating blame. This requires a cultural shift of some magnitude, coupled with sensitive handling. It should also be seen as working within an ethical and legal framework aimed at getting the best out of practitioners rather than penalising them when adverse events occur.

Principle 5 – processes should be strengthened and developed to allow for better identification of risk

Healthcare professionals are surrounded by data – they are data-rich, but information-poor. It is important not just to follow rituals by completing forms and writing reports, but to think about what this data suggests about practice and, more importantly, the risks prevalent in practice and how they can be reduced.

Incident reports, patient complaints and suggestions, legal claims, morbidity and mortality data, audit results, risk assessments and research findings are everyday tools of the trade for healthcare workers, but as yet are not fully utilised to identify problems and improve practice. Much can be done to integrate information and make informed decisions about the risks in practice when information is utilised to its maximum potential.

Principle 6 – managing risk is both a collective and an individual responsibility

People often say that 'the organisation should do something' when in fact the organisation is a group of employees working towards the development and delivery of healthcare. In many cases this phrase is used to define board-responsible officers, and is aimed at placing decision-making with them in order to allocate responsibility for perceived or actual failures. Individuals must recognise that there is individual as well as collective responsibility and this sense of ownership needs to be accounted for in the way an organisation approaches and introduces risk management. Whilst there is corporate responsibility, each individual also has a responsibility in law to identify risk and take steps to control it.

Principle 7 – recognise that resources may sometimes be required to address risk

Not all risk reduction is dependent on finance, but it may involve the application of human resources. To think that all risk can be reduced without some investment is not only unrealistic but naive.

Notwithstanding problems with financial constraints, lack of resources – particularly for safety matters – is not a defence in law. To counter this and retain a sense of pragmatism, it is important for staff to determine what risks are acceptable and what risks are not, through prioritisation. This cannot be done in isolation and must be done in an open and inclusive way.

Principle 8 – every organisation should strive to understand the causes of risk, its link with quality and the importance of addressing issues

Risk management is a learning process using methods to identify, assess and control risk. It has to form part of other approaches used by clinicians, staff and managers.

Causes of risk may stem from the way the organisation or practice is structured, the number of staff employed and their mix of skills, or alternatively from an absence of guidance or procedures to illustrate what is expected of staff. Risk may be linked to the physical or psychological environment, or individual factors such as behaviour, competency or supervision.

Addressing root causes is not just about reducing risk, but improving quality. These two concepts tend to be dealt with separately, but they should be seen in the same context. Clarity through information, education and development should help to lead the way and move quality and risk forward together.

Eight principles have been outlined, each with a summary of the issues that need to be considered and which should form part of an overall strategy for risk management, discussed later in this chapter.

Before this can be done, a step-by-step guide to risk management will now be discussed in order to give readers the tools to begin the process.

The process of risk management

Risk management is about the planning, organisation and direction of a programme that will identify, assess and ultimately control risks. It offers a framework which others can work to and operate within. The best way to illustrate this is shown in Figure 1.

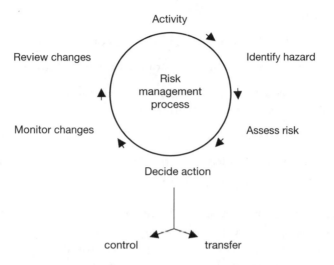

Figure 1: The risk management process

Every organisation has some level of risk, whether associated with medical treatment, financial planning, or the recruitment and retention of staff. Risk management is about bringing the risks from these activities together in order to allow risks to be viewed both strategically and operationally. This in turn will allow decision-makers to consider the quantity and extent of risk presented and to make some choices about them.

Types of risk

To begin with, an appreciation of the type of risk is required. There are two types: pure and business risk.

Pure risk

This consists of:

- physical effects of nature, such as floods, fire, or weather conditions

- technical issues such as breakdown of equipment

- personal issues such as sickness or injury

- social deviations from expected standards of conduct by staff – such as theft, violence or negligence

Business risk

Business risk differs from pure risk in that its components are:

- the impact of new technologies or changes in technology

- social impact, such as changes in expectations – for example, patients expecting better treatment

- economic impact such as inflation or budgetary constraints

- political impact such as the imposition of government ideologies, policies and philosophies

Pure and business risks can be considered as separate entities, but their inter-relationship is clear and should be acknowledged. As an example, a fire in a hospital or general practice would be classified as a pure risk. Depending on the extent and damage of the fire, it could have an impact on the finances of that organisation (hence business risk) due to a need to replace equipment and buildings, which could lead to an inability to treat patients.

Identifying hazards

In the previous section, risk and the understanding of risk was described and discussed. However, an understanding of hazard and risk is also needed so that a distinction can be drawn between the two.

Risk has been defined as the probability or likelihood that harm will occur and the consequences if it does. Hazard on the other hand is the ability to cause harm, the precursor to risk. For example, an electrical cord placed across a corridor is a hazard, while risk is the likelihood that someone would trip or fall as a result of it being placed there. By removing the cord, the hazard and the risk are eliminated. By covering the cord with a protective cover, the hazard is still present, but the risk is minimised.

The first step, as shown in Figure 1, is to consider the activities of an organisation – whether this is a precisely defined activity such as manual handling of equipment, or a wider activity such as surgery. Once the activity is identified, the process can begin. The next step is to identify hazards associated with the activity. Using surgery as the activity, some of the hazards identified are listed in Table 1 along with their potential effects.

Table 1: Hazards in surgery

Hazard	Potential effect
• Anaesthetic equipment	Harm to or death of patient if equipment fails
• Unmarked syringes	Wrong drug or dose resulting in harm
• Handling clinical waste	Possible infection from contamination
• Needles	Possible infection from needlestick injury
• Slip, trip or fall	Injury to body, such as hip, leg, back, head
• Use of disinfectants	Respiratory or skin sensitisation
• Moving patient on to table	Back or shoulder injury
• X-ray equipment	Over-exposure to radiation
• Blood or body fluids	Infection from exposure

Assessing risk

Identifying hazards can be relatively straightforward. It is determining whether a risk exists, and if so to what extent, that can be the most problematic. This is the assessment process. It is also the stage where human factors come into play because of the subjectivity a person will bring to the assessment process, even if a quantitative approach is applied.

The assessment process entails analysing the hazard and determining, based on the information and evidence available, the extent of the risk.

Quantitative versus qualitative approaches

This can be done using mathematical models – a highly quantitative approach – or much more subjectively using a qualitative approach. Either way, there is no right or wrong answer, nor should the conclusions be seen as binding for all time, but rather taken as a snapshot of what the level of risk appears to be at the time of assessment.

Risk is a moving target and is underpinned by a degree of uncertainty. Figure 2 illustrates a relatively simplistic approach to

17

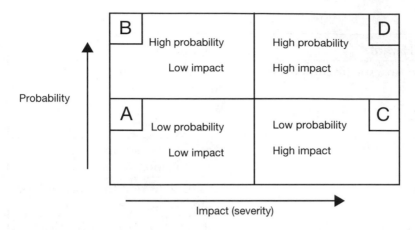

Figure 2: Probability and impact of risk

determining the level or extent of risk, using two parameters: probability and impact. Other assessment models also include frequency as a parameter, but for the purposes of this discussion, only the two will be used.

Let's take the practical example used before – the trailing cord. Depending on its placement and the environment, the level of risk will vary. Consider that the cord is attached to a floor-scrubbing machine used in a hospital corridor with a high throughput of people. It does not have a protective cover over it because the machinery is in use and is therefore mobile. It crosses the thoroughfare used by people visiting the hospital.

In this case the probability that someone will make contact with the cord is high (boxes B and D). The next consideration is what the severity of impact would be if a person made contact with the cord and fell. Most people would conclude that the impact would be high with some sort of identified injury; but would it?

The predisposition of the individual or group of individuals would need to be taken into account; for instance, would those likely to be affected be young, old, physically able or disabled? The impact on an older, frail person with poor mobility and osteoporosis would be much greater than on someone in their early twenties, who is fit with good balance. The severity of an injury to the older person could be much greater – for example, a fractured hip – but that is not always the case as chance plays a part. A younger person could begin to fall, place their hand out in an attempt to stop the fall and end up with a broken wrist. Nonetheless, a number of factors begin to come into play which can either be accounted for or ignored depending on how generic or specific the assessment is to be. Already the complexity of assessment is beginning to emerge.

Notwithstanding the complexities that arise, consider that a generic approach is taken and the extent of risk assessed is deemed high in terms of both probability and impact (box D). From this conclusion, we move to the next step: determining action.

Transfer or control?

In Figure 1 two paths can be taken – either controlling or transferring the risk. For the earlier example, transferring the risk could be an option – for example, contracting out the cleaning service and holding the subcontractors responsible for the safety of the systems they operate. But in reality, an organisation would aim to control the risk, even with a contractor, especially since the organisation will carry the liability under health and safety law for persons on the site. It could eliminate the risk, choosing to remove this area from the cleaning rota, but that would neither be acceptable nor particularly workable. Risk transfer is therefore not an option.

Options for risk control

The control of the risk could be varied as listed below and could incorporate a combination of options rather than just one, such as:

- scheduling floor cleaning for late evenings or over a nightshift when the number of visitors or others on the site is at its lowest

- installing additional electrical sockets so cords are not trailing across corridors

- replacing the flooring material with another that does not require this type of floor maintenance

- marking off the area where scrubbing is carried out with cones and warning signs, scrubbing one side of the corridor followed by the other

- introducing a cleaning system that does not require the use of floor-scrubbing machines

Cost/benefit analysis

The first three options carry more financial resource associated with either enhanced payments for nightwork, or installation of sockets or replacement flooring, but the cost should be set against the assessment of the risk. In essence, a cost/benefit analysis could be undertaken to determine which action would result in the more viable cost benefit whilst achieving the outcome of improved safety for those using the corridor. This can be a pretty fraught area to contemplate, but even if it is not accurate, it is useful nonetheless.

To return to the floor-scrubbing example, a possible conclusion could be that the worst case scenario would be for someone to fall over the cord, badly injure themselves requiring hospital treatment and then sue the hospital for not upholding their duty of care under health and safety legislation. This then needs to be set against the cost of moving the work to a nightshift or replacing the flooring with another type of material that does not require this type of maintenance. Readers will see that there are a number of assumptions in this cost/benefit analysis that could be challenged – for example, whether there would be a legal claim and its cost – but nonetheless cost and benefit should be explored where possible. It lends credibility to the process – but only if the method used is a valid one, in other words it has some statistical evidence and information to support it.

The language of risk

It is important at this stage to consider how risk is expressed. The floor-scrubbing example uses the words 'high' and 'low' to describe the assessment, the words painting a mental picture of how likely a fall is perceived to be. Other possible expressions we might use include 'minor', 'major', 'critical', 'untoward', 'serious' and the like. These words are open to interpretation and conjure up a range of perceptions for different people.

In everyday use, precise definitions may be irrelevant because general concepts are understood. However, when an incident does occur, the lack of a universally understood term can create problems within an organisation, initiating reactions and behaviours that in hindsight may have been misplaced. The opposite is also true. The language we use can act as a distraction from risks that are truly significant, with great effort applied to issues which are of little significance. It is important that when we come to developing a risk management strategy, later in this chapter, that we have an understanding of what specific terms mean and how they should be used (see DEFINING RISK AND EXPRESSIONS OF RISK, p33).

Monitoring and reviewing

The example of floor cleaning demonstrates how a number of options are generated through the process of assessment followed by a decision to take corrective action. Deciding what is the best course of action is by far the most difficult because of the uncertainty that may surround the decision. It is important that irrespective of what action is taken, the way the decision was made and the process used to inform it are transparent and understood.

Once a decision has been made about either transferring the risk or controlling it, the implementation of the decision should always be monitored. This is good management practice and fits in with the concept of assuring the quality of the process followed.

Decision-making in context

Using a different example, consider how reducing risk in one situation may increase risks in other areas. That means that taking decisions on controlling risk cannot be done in isolation, but must be considered within the context of what is happening elsewhere in the organisation.

Example: clinical waste storage

Consider clinical waste bags being stored in a small sluice area with equipment and dirty laundry. A health and safety inspection report confirms that this is bad practice and contravenes legal requirements because of the potential for contamination of other products in the sluice area from the clinical waste bags. The ward sister is asked to put secure clinical waste containers on the ward, large enough to hold a number of bags. However, because of limited space in the sluice, she is asked to put them in the corridor.

What issues have arisen from this example? Two immediately spring to mind: first, what is the extent of the risk of contamination of other products − is it real or theoretical? Second, what would the consequences be of storing waste bags in a container in a corridor?

Taking the first point, there should be an explanation of the extent of risk posed by the clinical waste bags. Is it a high risk and if so, in what regard? More importantly, placing containers in corridors in a ward presents a different risk, in particular the inability to evacuate patients efficiently in the event of fire. Obstructions in a corridor are a much higher risk than that posed by the clinical waste bags in the sluice if you look at it in a wider context. That is how risk should be looked at and evaluated – within the whole context of the environment. What other actions could have been taken to reduce any risk, comply with good practice yet not obstruct the corridor (see box)?

The clinical waste conundrum

Alternative approaches to managing the clinical waste storage problem are:

- having the clinical waste collection increased so that bags are not stored with dirty laundry and other products

- sub-storage areas installed between a number of wards so that waste can be collected and moved from the ward at scheduled times

- scheduling the clinical waste collection times before linen and laundry changes are done so as to avoid the storage of both products in the sluice at the same time

---

Organisation, environment, person

Monitoring takes on a very important role when risk is identified, assessed and controlled. There are three areas that should be borne in mind when monitoring changes, and also within the context of a risk management strategy. They are:

- **Organisation**: financial management, organisational structure, law, standards, culture, priorities and both external and internal influences

- **Environment**: support, workload, physical and psychological environments

- **Person**:
  - if a patient: their complexity of condition, communication and social factors
  - if an employee: their knowledge, skills, competency and mental health
  - if a visitor: their expectations and their unfamiliarity with where they are

This is best shown as an illustration:

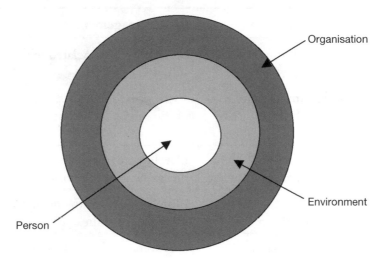

Figure 3: Risk in context

It can be inferred from this illustration that problems exhibited within the organisation will eventually have an impact on a person. Get the organisation right, and the risks can be minimised for others.

Risk and quality

One of the most important aspects of risk is to consider its link with quality, because risk management aligns closely with the principles of quality assurance. It can be said that risk and quality are interchangeable depending on how a situation is viewed – for example, reduced risk can lead to improved quality and vice versa. Table 2 (overleaf) describes how the two management systems relate.

One of the simplest ways of differentiating quality assurance from risk management is to think of quality measures as the outcome of a process, whereas risk management will concentrate on the input to a process, as illustrated in Figure 4 overleaf.

The discerning will see fault with this simple theory, noting that there are many assumptions inherent in this model, the first being that the risk is identified, known and without uncertainty and that using risk as the input, the outcome will be improved quality. How indeed is quality measured? If we revert to the clinical waste example, how would the quality be improved by moving the waste bags from the

Table 2: *Quality assurance and risk management*

Quality assurance	Risk management
Establish organisational goals	Identify risks associated with activity
Assess procedures in place to achieve goals of the service or activity	Assess risk as it affects all elements of the service or activity
Implement actions and measures to overcome problems	Develop and implement control measures to reduce risks
Monitor to assure desired result has been achieved	Monitor changes to ensure risks have been minimised
Document effectiveness of changes	Document effectiveness of changes

sluice into the hall? It could be that the space released in the sluice as a result of moving the bags has improved the quality of the environment, in other words it is less crowded and safer to work in. Not very measurable, but does it need to be? Perception can be enough, particularly if it improves morale.

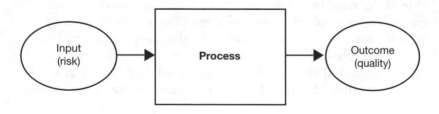

Figure 4: Risk and quality

Governance and risk management

Several related initiatives have been introduced in the years following the introduction of risk management. The first was corporate governance that arose out of a review of corporate business, known as the *Turnbull Report* (see KEY REFERENCES, piii). It focused on management ethics and a code of conduct aimed at increasing confidence in the way business operates.

From this report sprang clinical governance – taking the same concepts and applying them within a clinical setting – again in order to ensure there was transparency in the way healthcare was organised and operated and, importantly, to make sure that the public could scrutinise how the public sector operates. Two Department of Health policy statements in the late 1990s, *The New NHS: Modern, Dependable* and *A First Class Service* (see KEY REFERENCES, piii) outline the importance of quality and risk management and the need to have a governance framework to deliver improvements in health services.

Controls assurance

Controls assurance was first introduced to the NHS in 1999. This process, originally introduced for financial management, has now been extended to many of the functions of healthcare, such as medicines management and infection control. With its introduction has also come the challenge of another set of standards that healthcare professionals and managers are required to meet. Nonetheless, it is important to understand it in the context of risk management because risk management is a controls assurance standard itself (see Figure 5).

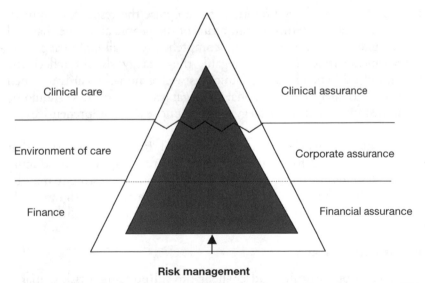

Clinical care   Clinical assurance

Environment of care   Corporate assurance

Finance   Financial assurance

Risk management

Figure 5: Controls assurance (Source: NHS Executive (see KEY REFERENCES, *piii))*

Risk management is seen as the glue that binds the functions of financial management, the care environment and clinical practice together. It is itself a function that can be applied to the financial setting, how the environment is organised and to how clinical care is delivered. The latter subject is discussed in more depth in chapter 4.

Each of the controls assurance standards has a number of compliance criteria. The standard on risk management looks at the capability within the organisation, the strategy and how it is implemented, what training and communication mechanisms are in place and, lastly, how a risk management strategy is monitored and evaluated.

Developing a risk management strategy

Developing a strategy in many respects is easy, it is effectively changing the way the organisation perceives and deals with risk that is the real challenge.

In developing a strategy, it is important to analyse what currently goes on in the organisation regarding risk management, followed by a critical analysis of gaps or improvements required. It is from this point that a strategy with clear aims and objectives can be derived.

Resources

During the process it is important to recognise the resources required, not just in financial terms, but in terms of the people and time that will be required to implement a comprehensive, all-embracing risk management strategy. In this regard, the strategy should reflect the breadth of risk, encompassing clinical as well as non-clinical issues such as health and safety, organisational and legal issues. All of these should be accounted for so that the strategy is clear, concise and comprehensive.

Risk management may require additional financial resources that must be accounted for. The arguments run parallel with introducing quality systems into an organisation where some investment may be required, but the gains at the end of the process are significantly higher than the original outlay.

A positive process

The biggest opportunity and challenge to introducing a risk management strategy is gaining the support and the hearts and minds of those in the organisation, to embrace and effect change. Risk management therefore should be seen as a positive process, not a punitive one and should foster a focus on learning, not blame. There should also be tangible outcomes for staff and patients to see – better clinical outcomes, an improved work environment and/or reduced stress levels for staff.

Purpose of the strategy

The purpose of a strategy is to determine the direction an organisation should be heading towards. In order to do this, three key elements must be in place:

- strategic analysis
- strategic choice
- strategic implementation

The corporate strategy model shown in Figure 6 can be used to help develop a risk management strategy.

Strategic analysis entails much of what was discussed earlier, so that an understanding is created of the political, economic and social environment in which healthcare operates. Whether it is general practice or a hospital setting, there will be influences that must be taken into account, such as legislation and DoH guidance. The

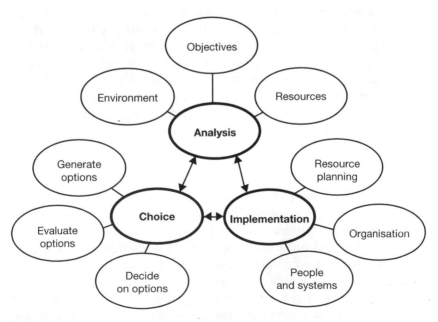

Figure 6: A corporate strategy model[4]

introduction of controls assurance standards is a further example. In addition, the healthcare organisation will need to look at the people, systems and resources that are in place to deliver its aims. This analysis should be as objective as possible and it must be informed. In essence, corporate strategy is looking at:

- where we are now (analysis)

- where we want to be (choice)

- how we get there (implementation)

Where are we now? Strategic analysis

Objectives

The review of where an organisation is in terms of risk management is the first and most crucial step in developing a risk management strategy. The purpose of such a strategy is to minimise and, if possible, eliminate risks to the organisation, the environment and people who may be affected. The expectations and objectives in place will, therefore, set the direction for the future.

Environment

Internal and external influences imposed upon and operating within the organisation will then need to be accounted for as part of the environmental analysis. It is important to be aware of and sensitive to what influences are about, taking account of them, but being mindful of the 'must-do's' placed on an organisation. The introduction of national service frameworks (NSFs) is a good example – the risk of not meeting the targets and quality standards within these must be taken into account when considering influences.

Resources

The third component of a strategic analysis should look at both financial and human resource. Who, for example, is going to lead the risk management process, at board level, at directorate level and within clinical and non-clinical services? Will the approach taken be based on everyone accepting responsibility for managing risk and in so doing, who will provide the leadership to drive the process forward? Trying to develop a risk management strategy without the resources needed will end in confusion with a job half done, and people not believing in the value of the work they have done.

Where do we want to be? Strategic choice

Generate options

Generating options can often be challenging and exciting, allowing people to express their ideas about how things can be done differently. Involving people is vitally important because it is the involvement of others that will not only generate the best ideas, but also instil a sense of worth and ownership in the process.

This does not mean everyone in the organisation has to be involved, but those people who have an understanding of the issues and of what could be done. This should encompass people from a range of professional groups, such as nurses, doctors, therapists, managers, technical staff, administrative and clerical staff. Together, they should formulate a series of options. This can be done in a number of ways, for example, through workshops, task groups, open meetings or small groups working by specialty. The more involvement they have, the easier it is to gain ownership of the strategy as it emerges.

Evaluate options

Once options for a strategic approach to risk have been identified, an evaluation of these options is required. This lends credibility to the process and sets the ideas generated into a realistic framework. This needs to be handled skilfully and with sensitivity, for once others are engaged in the process, it would be detrimental to all involved to then disillusion and isolate them through an evaluation process.

To avoid this, involve others in determining the criteria used to evaluate the options generated. For example, options might be generated ranging from doing nothing, to an option where a large number of committees and groups are established to work on specific risk issues. Criteria developed and applied to these options should include the amount of resources needed and whether the option generated delivers the best value for the organisation. Even by applying the latter criteria, subjectivity will arise and rightly so. As long as everyone is clear how options and thus decisions are made, then the process of evaluation will stand any scrutiny.

How do we get there? Strategic implementation

Once the choices have been presented and a decision made about a risk management approach, it can then be developed and implemented. To do this, three elements, shown in Figure 6 (p27), are needed: how the organisation is structured, what people and systems are in place and lastly, what resources and planning is required to put the strategy into place. A time element should accompany this stage of the process for it cannot all be done at once, but should be staged and evaluated as the implementation unfolds.

Structure and culture of the organisation

The structure and importantly the culture of the organisation are an issue for anyone introducing a risk management strategy. Much of this concerns identifying responsibilities. Risk management is indeed everyone's responsibility, as demonstrated through the *Health and Safety at Work etc Act 1974* as the most prominent example, but it is how the levels of responsibility are delineated that is important. For example, a nurse will be expected to identify, assess and control where possible risks to patients, the environment and staff. However, the nurse may not be in a position to solely control the risk because it may require additional resource over which they do not have authority. That does not negate the nurse's responsibility, but it does highlight the importance of having an organisational structure in place that is clear about levels of accountability and responsibility and where decision-making lies.

People and systems

The chief executive of an organisation has the ultimate responsibility for managing risk, leading the corporate responsibility with board directors. This applies in healthcare settings, with NHS trusts being the prime example. This responsibility is delegated on a day-to-day basis to managers within the organisation so that they are equipped to introduce a risk management strategy in a way that is inclusive, driven by those who provide care and that ultimately leads to changes.

Managers discharge their operational duties through the development of policies, procedures, guidance and protocols. It is the type of organisational rules that help bind an organisation into a structure that performs. Risk management is no different. Employees' responsibilities lie in working to the organisational rules that are developed and introduced, but also in their awareness of how they can influence and make a difference. This is the real change agent for managing risk.

Risk management strategy in practice

Thus far the corporate strategy model has been used to illustrate the process of setting about a strategy for risk management, but this has been confined to discussions based on models and theory rather than what really happens in practice. So how is a risk management strategy developed and introduced?

One way forward is for a group of individuals led by a senior manager to undertake the work as outlined in the corporate strategy model, in order to gain an understanding of how to set about introducing change within the organisation. There are six important ingredients that are required for a risk management strategy, even in its early development. These ingredients will set the tone of the strategy document and indicate how it will be introduced. These are:

Elements of a risk management strategy

1. having the support of the board
2. writing a strategy that is understandable
3. defining risk and expressions of risk
4. learning
5. communication
6. tools of the trade

---

1. Having the support of the board

It is nearly impossible to successfully introduce risk management into an organisation without the full support of the board. This support includes the chief executive, directors and non-executive directors. Because they are the ultimate decision-makers, if their support is not forthcoming, any risk management strategy will fail, no matter how good it is.

Therefore any risk management strategy must be developed with the visible and undeniable support of the board to the extent that is it is unquestionable. Assessment and inspection agencies such as the Clinical Negligence Scheme for Trusts (CNST) or the Health and Safety Executive (HSE) will require this, looking for a signature by the chief executive to a policy or strategy document as well as formal acceptance of it at board level. In addition, they will look for it to be in the public domain so that staff and members of the public are aware of the organisation's commitment to managing risk.

Having board support is all well and good, but there should be an appointed executive director with responsibility at board level for ensuring a strategy is developed and in place. This will vary according to the structure of the healthcare organisation. For example, in a large teaching hospital, the medical director or director of nursing will typically take the lead, usually as part of clinical governance. In a primary care trust, the lead may be one of the directors or alternatively the clinical governance lead. Irrespective of the type of healthcare organisation, there needs to be a named senior person who will voice issues at board level and provide leadership and support to others on behalf of the chief executive and management team.

2. Writing a strategy that is understandable

Strategy documents can be written in two parts, the background to the strategy and objectives, supported by a policy that sets out the operational procedures required to deliver the objectives. In this way a strategy can be confined to a few pages, with the policy and subsequent procedures providing the basis and detail respectively. The strategy sets the direction of travel, the policy outlines how the journey will be made, assigning responsibility in the delivery, and the procedures provide detailed instructions for each part of the journey.

A strategy should be written in plain English so that stakeholders can understand what its intentions are and, more importantly, how these intentions are to be implemented. In this regard, it is useful to have non-executive directors or lay people involved in its construction to avoid excessive management and clinical jargon.

A strategy should be realistic and not too ambitious, and should make some allowance for scanning the horizon for what is expected now and in the future. The strategy will provide a basis for short-term changes as well as longer-term ones, say over three to five years. Strategic documents should be subject to review with an acknowledgement that things may change due to external factors, but the essence of what is being achieved – reducing risk – will not.

3. Defining risk and expressions of risk

The document should provide a working definition of risk, similar to that proposed earlier in this chapter (see DEFINING RISK, p10). It should also give some guidance as to how terminology should be used and what it means. Don't forget the potential for confusion stemming from the type of language used, mentioned earlier (see THE LANGUAGE OF RISK, p20). It is preferable to work to common definitions used by the DoH for consistency and these should be stated somewhere at the outset of a strategic document.

4. Learning

The strategy should explain the philosophy of the organisation, its culture and how learning will be used to improve the quality of care and the reduction of risk. This is really about making sure the blame culture, if present, is eventually eliminated and, where it has been eliminated, to make sure it does not re-emerge.

Learning is the foundation for an organisation and the individuals within it to progress and move forward. Any good risk management programme should encompass learning as the platform from which to achieve its full potential. By adopting this approach, the strategy must therefore include teaching and training as a key element of the programme plus an effective communication plan that supports the whole of the strategy.

The strategy should include learning as part of an appraisal and personal development plan. In other words, each individual's responsibility in the management of risk should be part of their regular performance appraisal. Milestones for achievement, dependent on the job in the organisation, should be in their personal development plan. By using appraisal as a route map for learning, evaluation and changes in practice can happen in an informative and proactive way.

For medical consultants, one way of introducing risk management into their practice would be to assess, as part of their appraisal, how many clinical events they reported against the number of finished consultant episodes (FCEs) as well as the outcome of the events reported. It is the outcomes that are most important; addressing these ensures there is involvement by the clinicians in addressing risk and quality issues.

5. Communication

Communication forms an important part of the strategy document. For instance, what mechanisms will be used to communicate with staff, patients and the public about what needs to be done? It is unwise to invent complex mechanisms for selling the message. It is far better to use successful, tried and tested ones, exploring what methods of communication people are most likely to use.

Electronic communications systems

With an increased reliance on electronic communication systems in the NHS, one of the best communication tools is e-mail for key messages, supported by an intranet site that allows staff to find out what is happening and access websites for further information and learning. For example, the risk management strategy can be loaded on an intranet with hyperlinks to the DoH controls assurance website. Another, more innovative example is using clinical information systems such as pathology results electronic reporting, and presenting risk information through that medium. This can instil a sense of risk management with young clinicians who will be the people to take forward risk management in the future. To educate them as they progress through an organisation is one of the most enduring and successful communication strategies to apply.

Whatever communication systems are used, their effectiveness must be evaluated. There is little value in using a hospital newsletter to give vital information to staff if they do not read it.

6. Tools of the trade

Lastly, a strategy should set the direction for implementation, normally by giving staff a toolkit of ideas and guidance on how to proceed. For instance, the strategy might state that the tools needed to identify, assess and control risk are:

- incident reports
- complaints and claims information
- morbidity and mortality data
- clinical and non-clinical audit information
- risk assessments

- external reports by, for example, the NAO, HSE, CNST and auditors

The strategy should also establish the links between these tools and how the information will be used. Granted, some of this level of detail is more appropriate for procedure documents, but some indication of what is required to deliver change is necessary. It could simply be a statement in the strategy document that says: 'Risk assessment will be used to determine the extent of risk, supported by information from a number of sources, such as incident report data.'

Successful implementation

In summary, producing a risk management strategy can be straightforward provided the ingredients as listed are in place. However, do not underestimate the scale of the task in implementing a risk management strategy. The most important ingredient is communication. If the right message is given about what the strategy is, especially at board level, and it is backed up with learning, then the tools of the trade will fall into place. Make sure the support is there from the board from the onset and, over time, the strategy, its aims and objectives will be achieved.

Consequences of not managing risk

Not to put too fine a point on this subject, the worst consequence of not managing risk could be the death of an individual or several individuals. This could either be a patient under treatment or an employee who, as a consequence of poor risk management, is severely injured or dies. Readers will recall news stories where employees have been killed or severely injured in the construction industry or through other industrial processes. Every investigation or review of these tragic events shows weaknesses in the identification, management and control of risk.

The outcome of investigations in healthcare is not different. One only needs to utter the word 'Bristol' and immediately the children's heart surgery scandal (see KEY REFERENCES, piii) comes to mind. This is unfortunate because the standard of overall clinical care and treatment within this establishment was good, yet the damage done by this case will be with the trust for years to come. One consequence, therefore, of not managing risk is the damage done to an organisation's reputation and the lack of confidence that accompanies it, especially by its users.

Costs to the organisation

Time and time again the behaviour exhibited by individuals or companies, through short cuts, investments not being made or employees not being trained, culminates in some damage. One consequence is a loss of reputation and confidence in an organisation through the poor management of risk, which affects individuals in a number of ways, death, long-term disability and chronic health problems being the worst possible outcomes.

Another consequence of an organisation not managing risk as well as it should is increased costs, as illustrated in the box opposite.

Risk and the law

Another important consequence of poor performance is the recourse to the law for those who want retribution for what has happened to them. The increased projected costs of clinical negligence claims year on year in the UK point to a society that is more willing to seek compensation through the courts if dissatisfied.

A defensive approach

Whilst this trend is not nearly as severe as in the US, it is a worry nonetheless. The immediate reaction for organisations, particularly healthcare providers, is to become defensive in their practice. This defensive approach pushes risk management into a function that is seen as a way to protect doctors and nurses from litigation, rather than as a method by which to highlight and improve care. The CNST, despite its efforts to be seen as a positive force for good, is publicly committed to reducing the cost of litigation by employing risk management methods. This approach has led many in the healthcare field to see these standards as simply an exercise in protecting a hospital rather than what they should be seen as – standards established to improve the quality of care provided.

Nonetheless, the cost of litigation is increasing as a more consumer-driven society develops. The consequence to hospitals and independent practitioners is an increase in the insurance required to cover potential liabilities. For a large hospital, this can be quite

Two examples of poorly managed risk

Poor infection control management:

A hospital-acquired infection is diagnosed in a ward. Infection control measures have been developed, but are not followed by nursing and medical staff. As a result, the infection spreads and patients with a higher risk of infection due to their medical condition become infected. Because the organism is resistant to most oral antibiotics, patients have to be treated with intravenous antibiotics, presenting them with additional risks and incurring higher costs to the organisation. The length of stay at the hospital for these patients may be increased, and one consequence may be beds blocked for other patients.

Poor employee relations

One department within the hospital is showing a higher than average sickness/absence rate plus a number of unfilled vacancies despite a good rate of pay and no national shortage of trained staff in this field. A review of recruitment and retention information shows a higher than average turnover in staff. Anecdotal evidence suggests that the manager of the department has poor communication skills, does not delegate to others, refuses staff training and development and is quite difficult to work with. As a result, potential employees in the market will not apply for jobs, seeking employment at the neighbouring hospital instead. The consequence of this is a demoralised workforce for those who remain and a less than adequate service because of staff vacancies. To counter this, agency staff would need to be employed to ensure safe staffing levels – a financial drain on the department's budget – in addition to covering those who are sick or otherwise absent.

substantive. It is also lost money, taken out of clinical care and held to offset the unforeseen.

A leading approach to managing risk

As this chapter makes clear, a number of consequences can arise if risk management is not developed and introduced, and an organisation and its people can be exposed to damage. It is only through leadership, constant reminding and demonstration that managing risk will benefit all. This benefit can show up in increased productivity and a more confident and efficient workforce.

There is also a stark reality for those who take on the mantle of risk management and lead it in their organisation, and that is that this subject competes with many other pressing priorities in a fast-paced world. This is particularly true within the healthcare sector and it cannot be ignored.

This chapter goes some way to outlining a way forward for those wishing to embark on this journey, a journey which is well worth taking. Success lies in making risk management an integral part of the daily business of healthcare, not an additional bureaucratic burden aimed at preventing claims or seen as an imposition from above. It takes leadership, backed up by sound communication and negotiation skills by those involved. If these are applied, an organisation secure in how it operates, with a view of risk as a positive approach to improving practice, will emerge.

References

See also KEY REFERENCES, piii

1. Willett, AH (1951), *The Economic Theory of Risk and Insurance*, Irwin Publishers, Illinois, USA.

2. Knight, TH (1921), *Risk, Uncertainty and Profit*, Houghton Mifflin Company, New York, USA.

3. Bettis, RA (1982), 'Risk considerations in modelling corporate strategy', *Academy of Management Proceedings*, New York, USA.

4. Adapted from the work of Johnson, G and Scholes, K (1989), *Exploring Corporate Strategy*, Prentice Hall Publishers, Hertfordshire.

Further information

Berstein, PL (1996), *Against the Gods: The Remarkable Story of Risk*, John Wiley and Sons, New York, 1996.

Burrows, M (2000), 'Trauma care, a team approach', *Risk Management*, Butterworth Heinemann, Oxford.

Burrows, M (1994), *Risk Management Applications in Healthcare*, dissertation submitted to Leicester University.

Burrows, M (2000), *Consent to Treatment*, dissertation submitted to Cardiff University.

Carter, RL (1994), *Handbook of Risk Management*, Kluwer Publishing, Surrey.

Collis, D (1992), 'The Strategic Management of Uncertainty' *European Management Journal*, Vol 10, no 2, pp125–135.

Rockett, JP (1999), 'Definitions are not what they seem', *Risk Management, An International Journal,* Vol 1, no 3.

Rowe, WD (1977), *Anatomy of Risk,* Wiley Publishers, New York.

Wilson, C (1987), *Quality Assurance and Risk Management: Two sides of the same coin,* unpublished paper, Canadian Institute of Law and Medicine Fall Conference, Toronto.

Stalvies, C (2000), 'Taking a risk – and managing it', *Health Care Risk Report,* Vol 6, no 9, pp18–19.

3 Incidents: recording, analysis and investigation

Mary Burrows

This chapter covers:

- **Defining incidents**
- **Methods for reporting incidents**
- **Categorising incidents**
- **Analysing data**
- **Learning lessons from incidents**

Much has been written on the establishment of procedures for the identification, reporting and management of incidents, but little critical evaluation of the effectiveness of incident recording as a risk management process. Many readers familiar with incident recording will have experienced frustration with the associated bureaucracy, and the inability to learn lessons from the incidents that continue to occur.

Some of this may be a result of the reluctance of clinicians and managers to take raw incident data and analyse it to the extent that it yields valuable management information. Another complicating factor is the difficulty of differentiating truly high-risk incidents from the vast number of diverse incidents that may be reported in a complex healthcare setting such as an acute hospital.

This chapter will therefore discuss the importance and principles of incident reporting, analysis and investigation, how it can be applied in a healthcare setting, its role as part of a risk management programme and its value in terms of changing working practices. This should enable readers to:

- define what incidents are

- understand why incident recording is an important component of any risk management strategy

- develop an incident reporting programme that covers the recording, analysis and evaluation of data

- utilise incident information to influence change in an organisation and learn lessons

This chapter focuses on the wide range of incidents that may occur in the healthcare sector, so there can be a better understanding of what information needs to be collected to inform change in an organisation.

What is an incident?

Standard dictionary definitions for the word 'incident' define it as a definite or distinct occurrence, or an event. In this context and for the ease of the reader, incident and event are used interchangeably throughout this chapter. A good working definition for an incident is:

> "any unexpected event that has an actual or potential detrimental effect on a patient, employee, member of the public or indeed the assets of an organisation"

Not to be content with a rather lengthy definition such as this, people tend to separate clinical events from those that are deemed non-clinical, in other words, not having a direct impact on a patient or related to a patient procedure. Sometimes this distinction is unhelpful, and can lead to energy being misdirected at how to record an incident, rather than learning lessons from the incident.

Accident or incident?

Why not use the word 'accident'? Accident usually refers to an event where there has been some damage, either to a person or to property. It implies harm or injury and when this happens, employees normally complete an accident form. Incidents, however, are much broader in nature and may imply injury or may not. Therefore it will be assumed, for the purposes of this chapter, that all accidents will result in injury of some sort, whereas an incident may not. Hence the reason why 'incident' is the preferred word as opposed to 'accident'.

DoH terminology

The Department of Health has reiterated the importance of staff welfare and staff involvement in ensuring patient safety and has introduced a national system of reporting. The DoH has adopted different terminology, preferring 'adverse healthcare events' (AHCE) and a 'healthcare near-miss' (HCNM). These are defined as follows on p35 of *Building a Safer NHS for Patients* (see KEY REFERENCES, piii):

*   An adverse healthcare event is an event or omission arising during clinical care and causing physical or psychological injury to a patient.

*   A healthcare near-miss is a situation in which an event or omission, or a sequence of events or omissions, arising during clinical care fails to develop further, whether or not as a result of compensating action, thus preventing injury to a patient.

The definition is further expanded in *Doing Less Harm* (see KEY REFERENCES, piii). In this guidance an adverse patient incident is defined as "any event or circumstance arising during NHS care that could have or did lead to unintended or unexpected harm, loss or damage". These definitions are narrow as they only relate to patients, whereas in order to effectively manage risk, other types of incident, such as those involving staff, also need to be captured.

Irrespective of the terminology used, being able to define and then classify an incident is important if this information is to be used to assess and manage risk. Near-miss incidents or events are extremely important to capture as they tell the story of what might happen in the future. The three-incident rule is a good one to go by – if the incident or near-miss has occurred three times, there will be a likelihood that the fourth event will be of a serious nature, although, in reality, a more serious outcome could happen at any time.

Why do people fail to report?

The difficulty with incident reporting appears to be in the process itself, not because it is not straightforward, but because of how incident reporting systems are used. If we think about it, incidents are reported every day in a variety of ways – the accident seen on the road and the subsequent phone call to the police, the leak in the washing machine, the scorched shirt during ironing or the gift vase broken after a child's birthday party. We think nothing about telling others about these events. So why is it any different when we are in the work environment? Why is it that reporting of events, however insignificant, becomes something so difficult to do? It might be the theory of 'big brother', people's perception that the organisation is watching and therefore shouldn't know too much about what goes on. This might preserve autonomy from those in authority, in order to maintain some sense of control in the workplace.

However, what of incidents that must be reported because there is a legal requirement to do so? The *Reporting of Injuries, Diseases and Dangerous Occurrences Regulations 1995 (RIDDOR)* is a prime example of health and safety legislation that requires individuals and organisations to report certain categories of incidents. Yet time and time again it can be shown that despite the duties outlined in law, individuals and organisations continue to fail to report, more so out of ignorance or lack of understanding rather than malicious intent. Incident reporting is not seen as necessarily important or core to the business, when in fact it most certainly is.

Methods of reporting

Journals, textbooks and articles are strewn with information on how to report incidents – the use of forms, confidential telephone lines, in person, with or without a witness, by facsimile or through electronic databases. Then there is the question about which systems are preferable; for example, if a written form is to be used, then what design is required to capture relevant incident information? The question of what is relevant information arises – or, in other words, what is the necessary data set required? There is also the question of who should see the form once completed and who is responsible for taking any action following the incident.

Designing incident forms

Not surprisingly, opinions differ on all these aspects, often to the point of distraction. With forms, for example, some prefer free text, but others wish to use tick-boxes or checklists only. In addition, opinions differ about whether there should be one form for all incidents or separate forms for clinical and non-clinical events and even separate forms within these subdivisions. It has been known, for instance to have a form for clinical incidents, one for accidents, one for violence and one for drug errors. A system that is complex from the outset will struggle because of the demands it will make on those who have to use it. It is unlikely that with a number of different reporting systems that full reporting will take place.

For those that have had any experience of designing incident forms, they will attest to the difficulties that arise during what appears to be a pretty straightforward process. Discussions can become very emotive and highly charged, especially concerning where organisational logos will appear – everyone becomes a graphic designer when incident forms are being developed! To avoid this, here are some key points to remember when setting up an incident reporting system for the first time or alternatively, when a system is being reviewed.

Developing an incident reporting system

Research existing systems

Before beginning the process, research what is being done in the healthcare field on incident reporting. Gather information from similar sized healthcare organisations, for example, from a large teaching hospital, a district general hospital and a primary care trust. It is also useful to find out what type of systems general practice are using.

Then move on to explore what other industries, such as airline, railway and nuclear power, have done. These are all high-risk industries not unlike healthcare and they can offer a lot when it comes to designing a process used by thousands of employees. Not only should the research look at what systems they are using, but also what their future plans are for reporting, analysis and improvement of the system. It is also useful to consider the many incident reporting systems available as software packages. Most of these have not, however, been developed specifically for use in healthcare.

Set the research in context

This information should then be considered and set in the context of the organisation's work. For example, if the organisation is well advanced with computer hardware and software and has competent users, an electronic system for incident reporting is worth exploring. If not, then using a paper reporting system to begin with supported by a method of collating the data, normally through a database system, is preferable. A plan can be put in place to move to electronic reporting in future.

Explore alternative systems

Other methods should also be explored, for example, the use of telephone reporting and confidential or anonymous ways of reporting events, especially critical ones. Audit of medical records for determining any adverse event is a good way of identifying incidents retrospectively and can be used as part of a peer review or appraisal process. This information should be added to the research information already gathered, critiqued and an analysis done on the research to date. The aim of this is to be as well informed as possible prior to embarking on a project to set up both internal and external incident reporting.

External incident reporting

External incident reporting will be required in two ways, one as set out in law through *RIDDOR* and, secondly, through the requirements laid out by the DoH for the reporting of untoward incidents, sometimes referred to as critical events. External reporting will be discussed in more detail later in the chapter.

Involve a range of staff

When a reporting system is about to be devised, a range of staff should be involved. Healthcare professionals spend a considerable proportion of their day documenting information, so any increase in their workload through the introduction of another form must be done with care. They will have a clear view about what methods should be used, and this resource should be tapped into and used. Their ownership of the process and their involvement in its introduction will ensure the success of any incident reporting process.

One of the best ways to do this is to make sure a number of doctors' views are obtained during the development of a reporting system. Whilst nurses, therapists and other clinical and non-clinical support staff should be asked, so too should doctors for they are the one group of professionals that use the forms the least, yet are often best placed to report. Their input is therefore vital.

Keep it simple

There is nothing more frustrating than to be involved at length in the development and introduction of a complex system and then find it is seen as an imposition by management and therefore part of some political, externally influenced ideology. This is a view that has been expressed over a number of years by clinicians.

Clinical staff are focused on what goes on in their environment and want any system that is introduced to be one that will support them, not distract them from their duties, where possible. This has to be a critical factor when considering the introduction of a reporting system – keeping the system simple is a good principle to abide by.

Communicate

Make sure that everyone, as far as possible, is aware that research into and development of an incident reporting system is taking place, why it is being developed and what their role in it will be.

- Tell staff who is being consulted and seek volunteers throughout the process.

- Use tried and tested communication methods such as newsletters or team briefings.

- Make sure there is a contact person in case there are questions.

- Give an indication of when the system will be introduced.

- Conclude with what training and education will be available to staff in order that the system is successful.

Putting policy and ideas into practice

Incident reporting itself is not a means to an end, but a tool that can be used to reduce risk and improve working practices. It should not generate an industry in itself and must be seen as a spoke in a wheel rather than the wheel itself. To let it become an industry is to lessen the importance of incidents and how they can influence and change the behaviour of individuals or an organisation itself.

The purpose of incident reporting is to learn the lessons of past mistakes and change working practice so that further incidents are avoided. Changing the culture of the organisation so that incidents are seen as a positive indicator of performance as opposed to a negative one is the objective to achieve. In chapter 2, the organisation, the environment and the people involved were described as key to having an effective risk management strategy (see Figure 3, p23). These three factors will be used as the basis to show how incident reports and improvements in risk and quality are linked.

Demonstrating how incidents work within the scope of risk management is best shown using the example of a medication or drug error that occurs in hospital.

Case study: medication error

Setting the scene

Patient B has been given medication prescribed for another patient, patient A, who is located in the same bay (see Figure 1).

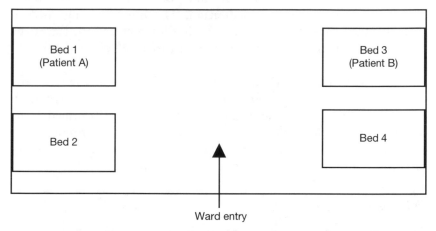

Figure 1: Ward layout for four patients

Patient A is located in Bed 1. Patient B is located in Bed 3. Due to staff shortages, a bank nurse is brought in to work the late shift. There is a policy in the hospital that any bank nurse has to be supervised in the checking of any medications, but if they have the appropriate experience, they can administer as part of a team.

At the nursing station there is a whiteboard with each bed number (there are 28 beds in all). Beside each bed number on the whiteboard is the patient's name and their assigned consultant.

All 28 beds are full with medical patients, and the average patient age is over 65. Some of the patients are very ill and therefore highly dependent on nursing care. On this particular shift, the bank nurse is assigned a number of bays with a particularly highly dependent caseload. There are two other qualified nurses on duty and one healthcare assistant.

What goes wrong

Medications are checked following procedure and the bank nurse begins to administer medication to patients in the first bay, numbered beds 1–4. The nurse checks the whiteboard for Patient A and the patient's location, satisfied that Patient A is in Bed 1. The nurse then proceeds with the medication to the bay, enters it and moves to Bed 3 rather than Bed 1 thinking that Bed 1 is on the right rather than the left.

The nurse approaches the bedside, quietly asks the patient in Bed 3 if they are Patient A. The patient nods their head and the nurse proceeds to administer the medication. The nurse, having checked that no other patients in the bay are due for medication, leaves the bay and documents the administration on Patient A's chart.

Patient B calls out shortly after and the healthcare assistant nearby goes in to see the patient. Patient B asks why medication was given when the patient was sure their medication had finished. The healthcare assistant speaks to the bank nurse and then, through their conversation, it becomes evident that the medication given was not prescribed and, in fact, was given to the wrong patient.

Establishing the mistake

The nurse notifies the senior nurse on the ward and as they retrace the steps up to giving the medication, it becomes apparent that two fundamental errors were made. These were:

- The nurse made an assumption about the arrangement of the beds, believing that Bed 1 was located in the upper right hand corner of the bay, when in fact Bed 1 was in the upper left hand corner of the bay.

- The nurse asked the patient their name, and they appeared to respond in the affirmative. What the nurse did not do was actually check the patient's wrist identification band to confirm identity.

This second action just compounded the initial error. Referring back to the scope of risk management, the incident can be broken down and examined as to what may have gone wrong and how it could be prevented again. In this way, reporting and analysing an incident can be productive and used as an educational tool. In addition it can also lead to changes that may prevent the incident from occurring again.

Analysing the incident

The people

Those affected in the medication error incident are four people: the patient who received medication in error, the patient who did not receive medication, the bank nurse and the senior nurse. In this particular case the patient did not sustain any adverse affect other than being a bit sleepy. The doctor was notified and observations were taken to make sure the patient did not suffer any ill effects. The error was recorded in the patient's medical record.

The nurse, as expected, was very upset and wary of proceeding with administration of any other medications on the ward. As a result, the senior nurse decided to supervise any further administrations, resulting in a delay for some patients due to the dependency and staffing levels on the ward.

The environment

What was the environment like at the time? From the case study described, it was busy with a dependent caseload of patients for the bank nurse. During a review of the incident, a number of issues were highlighted:

- The whiteboard with the bed numbers and patient names was not supported by an illustration of the bay layouts.

- The beds themselves were not numbered.

- The bank nurse normally works on another ward and was therefore unfamiliar with this particular ward.

- Due to patients being quite ill on the ward and the ward being busy, the bank nurse was not given any instruction as to the layout of the ward before starting the shift.

- The nurse did not check the patient identification band to confirm the patient's identity.

- The nurse relied on the patient to confirm their own identity.

The organisation

Organisational risks, discussed in chapter 2, include issues such as policy and procedures, and human resources – which would include recruitment and retention strategies, education and clinical supervision.

During the review of the incident, a number of findings concerning the organisation were exposed:

- Because of recruitment and retention issues, staffing is below the required level for the number and dependency of patients admitted. Therefore the ward manager has to rely on bank nurses (those employed within the hospital, but who are willing to work extra shifts) and/or agency nurses (those employed by another organisation that are contracted to work on hospital wards as and when required).

- There are no procedures in place to make sure that bank or agency staff working on the ward are given an induction into the procedures of the ward itself.

- There are no procedures in place covering clinical supervision and the administration of medication for this particular ward. Instead it is up to the discretion of the senior nurse on duty to decide whether the bank nurse can administer.

The incident itself is a good learning tool for improving practice and the application of procedures within the ward. It is important to use the incident as a learning tool, as indicated, rather than seeking to allocate blame for the error itself.

Determining the level of risk

Considering the incident described above, it would be easy to immediately classify it as serious or significant – in other words, one that had serious consequences for the patient. But did it? This is where the subjectivity of risk comes into play.

Had the patient been given a morphine-based medication that had the effect of lowering the respiration rate, then it could be concluded that the incident was serious. If the patient had been given a standard antibiotic with nil effect, then the incident could be graded as insignificant or of low risk. But what if the patient had been allergic to the antibiotic? The outcome could have been very significant, with the patient having an allergic reaction, or in the worst case scenario, dying. This illustrates why it is so important to prevent incidents such as medication errors arising, as the eventual outcome is left to chance.

By considering different potential outcomes from the incident, it can be used as a learning tool to see how one error can multiply in magnitude. Using incidents in this way allows risk management to be a tangible, positive influence in making changes within an organisation without fear of retribution from others. Making incident reporting and learning a positive experience will make it a very effective tool in reducing risks within the organisation.

Recording and reviewing data

Incident reporting can be a force for good, but is not always seen as that, as organisational culture plays a key role in how incidents are dealt with. In the example, if blame had been apportioned for the incident and a warning issued to the nurse, the outcome might have been entirely different. This type of approach discourages an open culture which encourages and facilitates the reporting of incidents.

Recording data

How should incident data be recorded if it is to be meaningful and of use to the organisation? The starting point will be to identify the minimum data set required for data collection.

Minimum data set

A minimum data set should be based on the principles of who, what, where, when, how and why the event or near-miss occurred.

- **Who or what was involved?** – identification of the person or persons affected or equipment or facilities involved.

- **What happened?** – a description of the incident itself based on fact, not opinion.

- **Where did it happen?** – the location of the incident and the clinical speciality involved.

- **When did it happen?** – time and date of the incident.

- **How did it happen?** – an explanation of how the event may have occurred based on an analysis of the event.

- **Why did it occur?** – this will take the analysis a step further to look at what the underlying or root cause might be and what factors may have contributed to the incident.

In addition, other information that should be included in the data set is any action that has been taken to deal with the situation and what level of risk is associated with the incident. Of course, incident reports should identify who reported the incident and when it was reported, as this often differs from when the incident happened.

When to report data

Staff should be encouraged, if not instructed, as part of a policy and procedure on reporting, to report as soon as the event unfolds or is known about. This will allow those involved to discuss the incident with a clear sense of what happened, making it easier to understand and evaluate the incident. It will also provide a named person to contact if further information is required, an important point if an investigation is required at a later date.

Form layout

The design of the form, although this can be fraught with problems, is actually very important if an incident reporting programme is to be successful as part of a risk management and wider clinical governance strategy. A sample incident form is shown in Figure 2 opposite as an example of how information can be recorded using a simple layout. This is a working example from a NHS trust, developed on the premise that it needs to be simple and easy to complete, especially for medical staff, yet capture the maximum amount of data possible. It is supported by a software system and a coding system that allows meaningful statistics to be obtained with minimal effort.

Who needs a form?

The example form in Figure 2 includes a minimum data set and allows for some evaluation of what occurred. Of course, any form will need to be supplemented with a procedure so that it is clear what information should be provided and why. This particular form is one side of A4 paper, but is self-carbonating in three parts for the following reasons:

- one form is retained in the ward or department as part of its own internal audit and review process

- one is sent to the risk management or quality department for processing

- one is sent to another department or speciality that may have been involved

Date:	Time:	Location and specialty/department:

Name:	If employee: Full time or part time? Hours worked: Absent for > 3 days? Yes/No

Diagnosis (for patients):   Consultant:

Type of injury sustained:

Describe what happened stating only fact, not opinion:

Reported by: Signature: Date:

What action was taken at the time?

Reported by: Signature: Date:

Any follow up action required and by whom?

Level of risk attributed: None Minor Moderate Major Catastrophic

Contributory factors:		Notification/actions:	
Environment	☐	Recorded in notes	☐
Team	☐	Patient notified	☐
Individual	☐	Occupational Health notified	☐
Patient	☐	Legal department notified	☐
Task	☐	Statutory body notified (such as HSE)	☐
Organisational	☐	Other:	
Institutional context	☐		

This document is for quality assurance purposes only and should not be filed in any patient notes.

Figure 2: Sample incident form

An example which demonstrates the importance of the third copy is a dispensing error that is not picked up in pharmacy, but instead is picked up on the ward. The form would be completed and the third copy sent to the pharmacy manager to assess practice and quality control as part of their internal review of incidents and procedures.

It is worth noting that the contributory factor categories used in the same incident form are taken from the work of University College London and the Association of Litigation and Risk Managers, who have published a protocol for the investigation of clinical incidents.[1]

Primary care

The beauty of this sample form is that it can be used in primary care – with a few slight changes such as the removal of the consultant name. This is one sector of the NHS that has not been engaged in incident reporting, whether for patients or staff, in the way that NHS trusts and, to a lesser extent, health authorities have been. Some of this is based on the different relationship that exists with primary care in terms of their independent practitioner status and the contractual relationship that exists with a health authority and, more recently, primary care trusts. Indications are that this is set to change. The first way will be through the changes to the NHS proposed under *Shifting the Balance of Power*,[2] with the abolition of health authorities and regional offices and a shift of power to primary care trusts with expanded duties and functions. The second will be as a result of the increasing recognition that there must be accountability within general practice in a manner that is consistent with other NHS providers and one that instils confidence with the general public.

Tick boxes or free text?

One disadvantage of the sample form in Figure 2 is that legibility can become an issue. If a form is used that has tick boxes for a host of potential incidents within different specialties, then the data form can be scanned and automatically entered into a computer database system. With free text forms, the information needs to be entered into a system manually. An example of how tick boxes can be used is shown in Table 1.

Table 1: Tick boxes

Specialty		Category of incident	
• Cardiac	☐	• clinical (patient)	☐
• Medicine	☐	• security	☐
• Clinical support	☐	• staff incident	☐
• Surgery	☐	• violence	☐
• Obstetrics	☐	• drug/medication	☐
• Accident & Emergency	☐	• other	☐
Type of incident		**Specialty specific (acute)**	
• delay in diagnosis	☐	• removal of wrong organ	☐
• health records not available	☐	• allergic reaction to drug	☐
		• history not taken or checked	☐
• adverse drug reaction	☐		
• defective medical device	☐	• blood sample cross-matched for wrong patient	☐

An inclusive form

There is nothing wrong with the tick-box approach, but beware that to make the form as inclusive as possible for those completing it, many choices will need to be included on the form. The reason for this is to avoid overuse of the 'other' category: it should not become the default category because the person completing the form cannot find the category or description they are looking for.

The form can also contain specialty-specific sections for mental health, ambulance services and primary care. Examples of primary care can be related to a number of services; for dental treatment, for example: the extraction of the wrong tooth; excessive bleeding following treatment; or death as a result of anaesthesia. For general practice: an unexpected death in the practice or clinic; abnormal cervical smears not reported to a patient; incorrect repeat prescriptions for a patient; and, again, delay in diagnosis.

Statistics gathered from badly thought through incident reporting systems, whether free text, tick boxes or a combination of the two, include a large percentage of incidents recorded as 'other'. The question will always arise as to what exactly these are and vital risk management information may be lost.

The DoH form

The Department of Health has recently released its pilot incident report form, which can be found in Annex A of *Doing Less Harm* (see KEY REFERENCES, piii). The form is simple, confined to free text and, as expected, contains some of the minimum data sets discussed earlier. To ensure confidentiality, patient details are confined to factors such as gender, age and ethnic group if known. Staff involved are also granted anonymity; their designation is the only requirement.

Confidentiality

This approach provides the level of confidence required for a national reporting system. After all, it can be difficult enough to get healthcare staff to use an internal reporting system to its maximum advantage and, in so doing, feel safe in reporting. To step outside the organisation and report to a National Patient Safety Agency must be done in a manner that will ensure staff safety and security is maintained, even in this day and age of advanced healthcare and increased public scrutiny.

Grading incidents

The grading or categorisation of incidents is very important as it provides information on the level of risk prevalent within a speciality, but it also allows the organisation to prioritise and concentrate on the key issues arising from reporting. As shown in the sample incident report form, five risk-grading categories are used: none, minor, moderate, major and catastrophic. The National Patient Safety Agency uses these definitions. How these are defined for impact and consequence is summarised in Table 2 (opposite).

Establishing reporting as an everyday activity

Reporting is the operative word here for the assumption is made that all incidents are being reported, when in fact they are not. Therefore, the focus of activity is centred on a small proportion of reported incidents, with the unknown, hidden risks not being accounted for and therefore not being addressed.

'Corridor conversations'

This is where the informal personal networks of healthcare professionals become crucial, for they often indicate where there are

Table 2: Grading of incidents

Descriptor	Actual or potential impact	Numbers of persons actually or potentially affected	Actual or potential impact on organisation
Catastrophic	Death, including: • unexpected death whilst under the direct care of a health professional • death of a patient on GP or health centre premises • suicide or homicide by a patient being treated for a mental disorder • known or suspected case of healthcare associated infection which may result in death, such as hospital-acquired infection	• many (>50), eg. cervical screening concerns, vaccinations	• international adverse publicity/ severe loss of confidence in the organisation • extended service closure • litigation >£1 million
Major	• major permanent harm • procedures involving the wrong patient or body part • haemolytic transfusion reaction • retained instruments or other material post-surgery requiring re-operation • known or suspected case of healthcare associated infection which may result in permanent harm, such as hepatitis C (*continued*)	• 16–50	• national adverse publicity/major loss of confidence in the organisation • temporary service closure • litigation £500–£1 million • increased length of stay >15 days • increased level of care >15 days

Continued

Descriptor	Actual or potential impact	Numbers of persons actually or potentially affected	Actual or potential impact on organisation
Major *(continued)*	• patient receiving a radiation dose much greater or less than intended whilst undergoing a medical exposure • rape (but only on determination that a rape has actually occurred, or the organisation believes there is significant evidence) • infant abduction, or discharge to wrong family	16–50	(see previous)
Moderate	semi-permanent harm (up to one year), including: • known or suspected healthcare associated infection which may result in semi-permanent harm	• 3–15	• local adverse publicity or moderate loss of confidence • litigation £50,000–£500,000 • increased length of stay 8–15 days • increased level of care 8–15 days
Minor	non-permanent harm (up to one month), including: • known or suspected healthcare associated infection which may result in non-permanent harm	• 1–2	• litigation <£50,000 • increased length of stay 1–7 days • increased level of care 1–7 days
None	• no obvious harm	not applicable	• minimal impact, no service disruption

Source: *Doing Less Harm* (see KEY REFERENCES, piii)

particular incidents arising within the organisation. These informal networks, which might be termed 'corridor conversations', should be treated with confidence. However, if a serious risk is identified and it is substantiated by evidence, then it must be made clear to those who are aware of the incident that it must be reported through the appropriate reporting mechanisms. To ignore the incident could be a breach of duty of care of patients and a possible failure to comply with health and safety law. The *Public Disclosure Act 1998* makes it possible for individuals to raise concerns, but if the organisational culture is right, this should not have to be initiated through a whistle-blowing policy, even though it is right and proper to have this policy in place.

Over-reporting

The challenge, therefore, is to make incident reporting an everyday activity within healthcare, even to the point of over-reporting. This has to be done in a culture that is open and honest about incidents occurring, how they are reported and, more importantly, how they are dealt with and what lessons are learnt. To achieve this, there will be merit in having 'noise' in the system to begin with, through over-reporting, and then, through review and analysis of information, determining what the level of reporting *should* be. To do this will require a level of staffing that can cope with a high volume of reporting, provided the introduction of the incident reporting system is successful.

Reviewing incidents

'Review' of incidents is a positive term used for investigating an incident. The word suggests an approach that is open and transparent. 'Investigation' can often be taken to mean a harder-edged approach, even if it is not meant to be. Reviewing an incident fits in with the concept of risk and quality being interrelated in risk management, making it a positive approach to improving care rather than a negative one.

This is not to say that a review cannot be firm in its approach and searching within the process adopted. The Commission for Health Improvement undertakes reviews, and its published findings to date have had some far-reaching implications for NHS trusts. Depending on the type of healthcare organisations involved, reviews can be quite a useful tool to understand the root causes of incidents, and develop learning for staff and patients.

The review process

In reviewing incidents, there must be a person or persons responsible for managing the review, whether at a local level or at a wider organisational one. Incidents that are defined as catastrophic or major will certainly require a review. This should apply to near-miss events, not just those with a known impact or outcome, but also those where there is potential for harm as well. There must also be a clear procedure about what information will need to be gathered, what should be retained and the legal status afforded to the review and subsequent documents and reports.

Spotting incident patterns

Normally a clinical or department manager will undertake the initial review and in practice, senior managers get involved only if the incident is of such a serious nature that a wider review and analysis is required. An example of this would be the three incident rule, referred to earlier (see p42), where an incident is repeated three times but not necessarily by the same people or department. This trend would only be picked up by senior managers who reviewed reported incidents in a particular speciality, or those who review the data from the organisation as a whole and see the pattern emerging. This takes a keen and experienced eye.

Notification to outside bodies

Managers will also need to be aware of those incidents that are deemed to be critical or untoward and require immediate notification, both within the organisation and outside it. Outside notification is usually to the appropriate NHS regional office in accordance with their policies and/or to the Health and Safety Executive because the incident falls into the statutory reporting required under *RIDDOR*. After January 2002, adverse patient incidents falling into a high-risk category, as outlined in the guidance by the National Patient Safety Agency, will need to be reported to the agency using its patient incident report form. Procedures will need to be in place that outline the expectations and requirements of staff in this external reporting process.

What the review examines

Incident reviews will encapsulate the reason or reasons why the incident occurred. This entails looking at the level of performance of those involved and the environment at the time. Root cause analysis or similar methodology can be applied to identify and understand the underlying causes, including those that have an organisational origin.

Reviews may be seen as time-consuming in some cases, but they should nonetheless be recorded as part of the quality cycle of performance for a department, general practice or clinical speciality. Methods can be devised that make the process rigorous and thorough when it needs to be, but less thorough for low-risk incidents. One way to do this is by using the incident form as the review tool itself. Where a thorough approach is required, the use of an aide memoire or checklist can be used to guide staff through the process. For example, just a few of the things to be considered when undertaking a review are:

- reviewing documentation
- interviewing staff
- obtaining statements
- meticulous note-taking

Support for individuals

Where statements may be required, particularly if the incident may result in a potential legal claim against the organisation or an individual, staff should be given the opportunity to have a representative involved, for example a trade union official or personnel officer. This is vitally important to make sure the individual involved in the review is well-supported and is given access to essential information when needed.

The report

At the end of the review process, a report should be written that gives those involved an opportunity to comment on the findings. The report should:

- be concise and outline the key points of the review with supporting recommendations
- reference key documents that support the findings and recommendations
- give guidance as to what future changes will be required
- provide a timetable for putting in proposed changes
- outline who is responsible for ensuring that the changes are implemented

All reports should form part of a quality assurance cycle. This way there is a method of accountability to make sure that recommendations are indeed acted upon. One way of doing this is through the workings of a clinical governance and risk management committee. This will in part ensure senior management and board-level responsibility for incidents and risk.

Analysing data

Analysing information can often be the most challenging part of a review, but it can also substantiate the gut feelings of those involved. However, it can be difficult and confusing for a number of reasons. For example, there is too much information and those analysing the data may not have the skills necessary to discern what is important to focus on. Another reason may be the way the information is collated, which does not allow for particular patterns or trends to be identified.

Data should also be looked at in the context of other information and not in isolation. Incident reporting should therefore be seen as part of an information management system drawn from a range of sources and presented in a way that summarises the key issues and states assumptions where assumptions are made.

Analysing the data in context

The range of information sources that should be considered, compared and contrasted with data gathered from reported incidents is listed below. This list is not exhaustive, but gives a fair indication of information that can be used to obtain a picture of what is happening within the organisation. This includes:

- complaints information – generated by patients themselves or their relatives (this information is often complementary to incidents, and indicates when incidents should have been reported through the incident reporting system rather than as a complaint)

- review of medical records to establish any adverse events (usually through clinical audit cycles)

- morbidity and mortality data and peer review information

- clinical audit reports and recommendations

- potential claims held within the organisation

- claims data held by the NHS Litigation Authority – this can be used as a benchmark for levels and types of claims and give an indication of where incident reporting may be weak or ineffective

- reports from sources such as the Medical Devices Agency, the Health and Safety Executive and the National Audit Office

- regional information on critical adverse events notification and the National Patient Safety Agency

- stakeholders' views on the standard and quality of service

- assessments for the Clinical Negligence Scheme for Trusts and controls assurance

- Commission for Health Improvement reviews

Communications systems

Reviews of data in some healthcare organisations have shown that there is evidence of a correlation between incidents, complaints and claims but that to make effective use of the information, there must be good communication between people and services. If computer software systems are being used, it is preferable to either link these or use software that has the modules for each of these functions. That way one patient or employee database can be used, allowing an analysis of individuals as well as incidents.

Making the most of the data

So far the review of an incident has been considered on a case-by-case basis. From a departmental or speciality view, this is quite effective; but what do incidents say about the management of an organisation as a whole? The aggregation of data enables managers to determine what trends and patterns are occurring with reported incidents, and also provides a means of comparison with other organisations to determine what incidents are not being reported. It will be a requirement of the National Patient Safety Agency to provide incident information on a routine basis, excluding that required via their reporting form and system.

Essential functions of a data collection system

Whatever the data collection system used, certain information will need to be presented and commented upon. This is best achieved by using an electronic recording product, whether this involves commercial software or the development of an in-house database system. There are some essential functions that any system, even a manual one, must have if it is to provide useful management information.

These are:

- type of incident
- number of incidents reported
- contributory factors
- risk grading
- nature of the harm recorded
- location or speciality

1. Type of incident

This will give information on what type of incidents were reported. For example, how many were classified as clinical incidents, how many were non-clinical (which would involve estates and facilities issues) and, importantly, how many were classified as near-misses? Each type of incident should then be capable of being broken down – for example, clinical incidents would be subdivided into categories such as anaesthetics, surgery, treatment and diagnosis. Therefore, the coding system used within the organisation must be well thought through and lend itself to providing useful and meaningful management information.

2. Number of incidents reported

Just like information on complaints presented to trust boards, incident information should also give basic information such as the number of incidents reported over a specified period of time. This is normally shown quarter by quarter. The data can then be compared against each subsequent quarter or compared to the same quarter of the previous year or earlier, as shown in Figure 3 opposite.

Figure 3 demonstrates an increase in reported incidents year on year, with some fluctuation within the quarters of each year. This increase lends itself to various interpretations. One person may think that more incidents are occurring and thus there is an increase in risk within the organisation. However, another view may be that more incidents are being reported, but not necessarily occurring – in other

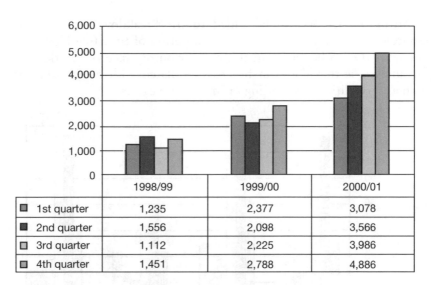

	1998/99	1999/00	2000/01
◪ 1st quarter	1,235	2,377	3,078
◼ 2nd quarter	1,556	2,098	3,566
◻ 3rd quarter	1,112	2,225	3,986
◩ 4th quarter	1,451	2,788	4,886

Figure 3: Number of incidents per quarter over three years

words, staff are actually using the reporting system, one small indicator that it is successful.

That is not the full story, however, because the numbers alone are meaningless. If the numbers were then taken as a ratio against the number of finished consultant episodes (FCEs) or outpatient attendances, then they would become more meaningful. It would also be much easier to see if there is a true trend in upward or downward reporting and there would also be an indication of whether the activity of the hospital in this case has increased or decreased. The HSE produces annual accident statistics which are expressed in frequency rates, that is, numbers of accidents for so many employees. This enables comparison to be made on performance across sectors.

3. Contributory factors

Not only is it important to classify the type of incident and establish whether the numbers are on the increase or not, but it is important to understand, through coding, what the contributory factors may have been. Referring back to the sample incident form in Figure 2 (p53), these are shown in the bottom left hand corner of the form. These contributory factors are usually determined during the review stage of an incident, but in the case of the organisation that uses this form, they form part of the incident reporting procedure.

Contributory factors can be added to the breakdown of incidents reported in a medical directorate over a period of time (see Figure 4), but what is even better about using contributory factors as a data set for analysis is that they can be cross-tabulated with other data sets such as specialities, risk grading or immediate causes.

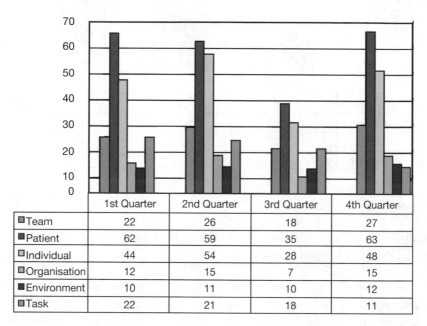

	1st Quarter	2nd Quarter	3rd Quarter	4th Quarter
■Team	22	26	18	27
■Patient	62	59	35	63
□Individual	44	54	28	48
□Organisation	12	15	7	15
■Environment	10	11	10	12
■Task	22	21	18	11

Figure 4: Contributory factors plotted against incident numbers

4. Risk grading

Working with the National Patient Safety Agency's recommendations and the risk grading shown in the sample incident report form in Figure 2, analysis of this data set is also of value. As a word of caution, however, (that should also be applied to contributory factor coding) the people applying the codes must be clear and consistent in the coding they use. If they are not then the data will not be useful, and can in fact skew the information in such a way that incidents requiring action are excluded.

5. Nature of the harm recorded

This will detail the injury sustained, if it is known at the time. This would include death, physical injury to parts of the body, pain, incapacity or disease.

6. *Trend analysis*

It is important to be able to break any recorded data down into the number and type of incidents reported by department, specialty or by practice, in the case of primary care. Comparisons can be made on a quarterly or other specified time frame and between specialties where there are common criteria, for example, the number of needlestick injuries sustained by nursing or medical staff or the number of back injuries reported. There must be caution applied when using this approach and a clear understanding of the criteria used to make comparisons. Any assumptions made must be clearly stated.

Other data sets can be used, such as incident costs, but these in the past have been often difficult to ascertain and use with consistency. There may also be an associated perception that incident reporting becomes more of a financial model for managing risk than a quality-driven one.

Electronic systems

It must be obvious that having electronic collection and analysis of data is by far the most preferable means of understanding incidents. To take this one step further, with the advancement of NHSnet and trust intranet systems, it is hoped that many paper-based incident reporting systems will move to purely electronic systems in due course. There would be a learning curve to overcome at first, but electronic systems have advantages over systems that operate a paper-based system followed up by entry into a commercial database system.

Benefits

The benefits of electronic entry include instant access to information and shortening the time of review and action, where needed. Such a system also gives clinical managers the ability to interrogate and analyse information from their own workplace, giving them the freedom and flexibility to be more proactive in managing risk in their own environment. Increased use of electronic-based systems also makes benchmarking easier.

In addition to the basic analysis of data, cross-tabulation allows the comparison of one data set against another to see if there are trends or patterns emerging. For example, contributory factors could be tabulated against a number of specialties to see if the individual factors were the most common factor involved in incidents reported. This would indicate, from an education and learning perspective, that support and supervision may be required in a number of areas. This can be broken down further to look at the professional groups involved.

Cross-analysis

The use of cross-tabulation produces a detailed analysis. It allows individuals to consider the information in a number of different ways and from a number of different angles. How the information is interpreted then becomes important from a management perspective.

Of course, all data recorded over time will bring the opportunity to map out trends. Through cross-analysis, however, this can be done in a more detailed manner. This could mean looking at clinical incidents on a month-by-month basis in one speciality, using the ratio figure rather than the raw numbers (see earlier discussion on the use of FCEs, p65) and tracking if there is a trend emerging. Good software packages or the application of the statistical analysis tools in a database package will calculate mean and standard deviation, regression lines and straight line extrapolations. The organisation will need to have people with good research and analytical skills in order to take this data, analyse it and present it as management information.

Learning lessons

Learning lessons from recorded incidents cannot be discussed without reference to the significant work undertaken for *An Organisation with a Memory* (see KEY REFERENCES, piii). This document paints a picture of optimism in the face of traditional ways of working and an NHS culture that needs to change. This change means NHS organisations becoming more open and transparent as public bodies and, in so doing, accepting their accountability to stakeholders. The NHS must be willing and able to admit to mistakes when it needs to, and to learn lessons from events.

This is of course easier said than done. High profile cases such as the Bristol paediatric heart surgery scandal, which resulted in an intensive public inquiry (see also chapter 9), and the Alder Hey Children's Hospital organ retention scandal have led the public to openly question the culture of the NHS, and rightly so.

A proactive approach

A much more proactive approach to identifying what goes on in a healthcare organisation, irrespective of its size, must be a good thing.

The concept of size is important, because media focus is often on acute medicine, the treatment received in hospital, or on a handful of cases involving mentally ill individuals. What it has not focused on is primary care, where the majority of first contact with the NHS takes place. Acute or secondary care is far more advanced in establishing a risk management strategy that uses incident reporting as one of the key tools to reduce risk and improve the quality of care for patients. It could be argued that the risks are not as great in primary care, but that could and should be challenged. Missed or delayed diagnosis, or inappropriate treatment and care, are just as important in the health centre or general practice setting as they are in secondary care.

Learning lessons across organisational boundaries

This leads to the consideration of learning lessons from incidents across NHS and social care boundaries. Both this chapter and chapter 2 imply that the systems to be put in place are only for a specific organisation, be it an acute care hospital, a doctor's surgery or a small community hospital. That is usually the case.

If the care provided is to be person-centred, then from the patient's perspective, who provides the care is irrelevant. What they are interested in is receiving the right treatment by the right people at the right time. If an incident occurs which disrupts the quality of that care, and if it occurs in more than one NHS organisation, how are the lessons learnt by all those involved? The answer is that at the moment, they are not.

With this in mind, this last and final section of this chapter will consider how lessons can be learnt, and, more importantly, that they must be learnt without the constraints of organisational boundaries. This does not just mean NHS boundaries, but also the boundaries between social care and healthcare.

Breaking down barriers

From a practical point of view, how are lessons learnt from reported incidents? The first step is to recognise the barriers to learning. Once identified, these can then be broken down and removed in order that effective learning can indeed take place.

Recognising personal fallibility

The barriers to learning are many and they apply to a range of organisations and industries, the NHS being no exception. The difference for the NHS is that the professionals it employs have a duty of care to others, both ethically and legally, that they must comply with. So one of the first barriers is the inability for professionals to recognise that they are fallible, can make mistakes and therefore have a need to improve their own practice and performance.

This first and profound barrier is actively being dealt with through professional bodies, but also by the Department of Health through the introduction of the NHS Plan (see KEY REFERENCES, piii) and the requirements that it imposes on professionals, from appraisal through to patient involvement and participation.

Ineffective communication

Another key barrier and undoubtedly one of the root causes of most incidents is ineffective communication within an organisation. This can be prevalent within clinical teams and at board level. Both can be damaging and can bar effective learning for many within an organisation.

Lack of corporate responsibility

Not having a sense of corporate responsibility is a barrier that makes it difficult to implement changes in behaviour and changes in practice. This could be particularly true with independent contractors who may not feel any corporate responsibility to a health authority or primary care trust because of their status. However, the same lack of corporate responsibility can also be found in district general hospitals, where clinicians opt out of decisions taken by the organisation and carry on irrespective of what has been decided or implemented.

Apportioning blame

Apportioning blame, a feature of inward-looking organisations with a very hierarchical and often dictatorial style, is another barrier that needs to be removed and replaced with a culture based on learning, not on blame. This requires leadership and very effective change management strategies employed over a period of time, and it may take years to see any demonstrable change. The time needed for this change, however, should not be an obstacle in itself to dealing with the issue of blame.

Individual reactions to criticism

The last barrier mentioned here (although of course there are more) is the difficulty that individuals have when faced with initiatives and the possibility that people will review and perhaps question their individual practice. Reactions to this vary, with some individuals finding it very difficult to listen to constructive criticism and others focusing on the process of incident reporting and the insignificant rather than the significant.

A learning organisation

Having dealt with barriers, or at least some of them, a strategy of organisational learning can begin. Learning is not simply about taking someone out of their environment for a training session, but using personal experience and learning as part of overall learning within an organisation. In addition, education and research must be the foundation for building a learning organisation, one which can continuously move forward to improve care.

These may be fine words, but the challenge is putting them into practice. By using some of the practical points outlined within this chapter, the foundation for learning can start to be applied, but this should be done in the context of other systems and procedures in place. There is a plethora of information available in healthcare settings and it is not used to effect.

Putting in a robust yet simple incident reporting system that can be integrated into operational activities is the first step, but it must be based on inclusion and consultation of staff. This way employees will feel they too have a stake in the system, are mindful to use it, and want it to be successful. Secondly, collecting the data in a clear and concise way and then presenting it as useful management information will allow the factors contributing to the incident to be exposed.

Taking this one stage further, aggregating the data and comparing and contrasting it both internally and externally, linking it with other information and devolving responsibility within the organisation to review incidents as part of a quality process will help achieve improvements and changes in practice.

Learning cannot be confined within the boundaries of one NHS organisation, but it must cross NHS and social care boundaries. If incidents are picked up in secondary care that may have originated in primary care, then it is feasible to discuss the incident with those involved and seek action to ensure that the incident does not occur again. Learning should be done in a way that is not threatening and is seen as an aid to improve care, focusing on the patient rather than on the healthcare organisation and its individuals.

References

1. University College London & Association of Litigation and Risk Management (ALARM), *A protocol for the investigation of clinical incidents*, Royal Society of Medicine Press, London, 1999.

2. Department of Health (2002), *Shifting the Balance of Power: the next steps*, (*www.doh.gov.uk*).

Further information

See also KEY REFERENCES, piii

Burrows, M (1997), 'Incident reporting and performance management', *The Healthcare Risk Resource*, Vol 1, no 2.

Department of Health (2001), *A Commitment to Quality, a Quest for Excellence*, (*www.doh.gov.uk*)

Health and Safety Executive (1997), HSG 65, *Successful health and safety management*, (*www.hse.gov.uk*)

Tingle, J (2000), 'The report that rocked a nation', *Health Care Risk Report*, Vol 6, no 8, pp 20–21.

4 Managing clinical risk

Jo Wilson

This chapter covers:

- **Clinical risk management strategy**

- **How clinical risk arises**

- **Active, latent and systems failures**

- **Risk factors highlighted by analysis of UK litigation**

- **Reform of the clinical negligence system**

- **The Clinical Negligence Scheme for Trusts**

- **Root cause analysis and risk modification**

The importance of the control of risk has been recognised by healthcare professionals for many years. In practice this is achieved by risk awareness, risk identification, review of practice and ongoing evaluation. Clinical risk in its simplest form is the potential for unwanted outcome. This is a very broad definition – it ranges from dissatisfaction on the part of patients or their families at having to wait too long for treatment or at a lack of communication, to undergoing the wrong operation, or suffering permanent disability or death.

From the patient's point of view, the risk of personal injury or disability, with the consequences for themselves and their family, is of paramount importance. However, for the healthcare organisation other consequences stem from an unwanted clinical outcome (see box overleaf). Each of these are associated with financial costs and decreased quality, which can place providers at a distinct disadvantage within the healthcare system.

Effects of unwanted clinical outcome

- extensive resource utilisation to correct the injury

- decreased productivity because of the time and resources spent in clinical negligence litigation, and incident and complaint investigation

- a tarnished reputation

- clinical liability awards to injured parties and legal costs related to the litigation process

- patient dissatisfaction

- locum cover costs and reduction in the quality of care delivery

- resource costs of facility downtime and improvements to facilities, and of public relations to improve local and public perceptions

Clinical risk management strategy

As outlined in chapter 2, a risk management strategy provides the framework for developing a rigorous risk management process throughout healthcare organisations. Further to this, each directorate or division should have its own clinical risk management strategy that links into the overall organisational risk management strategy.

The strategies should acknowledge that although healthcare is a risky activity, it is of considerable concern that a wide range of untoward incidents can occur by accident, mishap and mistake. Even more worrying are those which result from a lack of clear policies, procedures, protocols, care pathways, deficient working practices, poorly defined responsibilities, inadequate communications or other systems failures.

A proactive approach

The challenge for managers, clinicians and all other staff within healthcare organisations is to eliminate, or at least reduce, the potential for such misfortunes by being more proactive in the management of risk.

A clinical risk management strategy should include the following elements:

- a clinical risk management policy statement

- organisational arrangements for managing clinical risk
- the aspirations of the directorate or division concerned
- processes for identifying and assessing clinical risk
- key clinical, environmental and other risks to be addressed
- systems for preventing, containing, and controlling clinical risk
- use of clinical risk assessment tools, instruments and techniques
- arrangements for assuming, funding or transferring risk
- training and education requirements to make the clinical risk management process effective
- involvement of staff in identifying and managing clinical risk
- effective near-miss, incident and clinical indicator reporting systems
- management of legal claims and complaints
- monitoring of the risk management process

Focus on quality improvement

Clinical risk management must be seen as an essential component of an organisation's continuous quality improvement programme, embracing good working practices, processes and systems. A key to successful clinical risk management is to embed within the organisation the routine collection of relevant information, its analysis and the subsequent feedback to and assignment of appropriate action to clinicians and managers. Positive outcomes for clinical risk management are only possible where staff are engaged in the process and are given time and opportunity to reflect on their practice and take any necessary action to improve.

Central to success is the desire at board level to deliver services with minimal risk for patients and clients, and provide a healthy and safe environment for the organisation's staff. The board should also be aware of and comply with its legal and statutory obligations. To facilitate the risk management evaluation process, the healthcare organisation must prepare a comprehensive annual report of clinical risk management activities, and an evaluation of progress in this area.

An Organisation with a Memory

The clear message of the Department of Health report *An Organisation with a Memory* (OWAM) and *Building a Safer NHS for Patients* (see KEY REFERENCES, piii) is that in the past the NHS has failed to learn from mistakes. Adverse healthcare events are replicated again and again, but can be avoided if the lessons of experience are properly learnt. Clinical governance can provide a powerful imperative to focus on tackling adverse healthcare events.

OWAM report

To support this process and to modernise the NHS approach to learning from failures, the report calls for:

- unified mechanisms for reporting and analysis when things go wrong

- a more open culture, in which errors or service failures can be reported and discussed

- mechanisms for ensuring that, where lessons are identified, the necessary changes are put into practice

- a much wider appreciation of the value of the systems approach in preventing, analysing and learning from errors

All incidents should be viewed as free lessons,[1] and as opportunities to improve the quality of service provision. Incident reporting, investigation and follow-up are considered a minimum, level one standard of the Clinical Negligence Scheme for Trusts,[2] and alongside the complaints procedures provides a means of assessing areas where improvements need to be made. An open, just, honest and participative organisation, which aims to improve processes and systems of care, is a big step towards getting staff committed to quality.

Understanding the causes of failure

OWAM deals with the causes of failure – both human error and systems failure. Much work has been undertaken on these different approaches by Professor Brian Toft[3] and these have been applied to healthcare by Professor James Reason.[4]

Individual failures

The person-centred approach tends to dominate healthcare settings, leading to naming, blaming and shaming. Healthcare professionals adopt this stance among themselves and patients increasingly believe that if something goes wrong or there is an unexpected outcome, then someone must be to blame.

However, incidents almost always involve a systems failure – usually the combination of several factors coinciding. It is rare that there is only one person alone who is responsible, and blame that is applied is due more to opinion than fact.

Research undertaken by Professor John Overveit 1998,[5] demonstrates that 85% of incidents are due to organisational failures and 15% due to individual failures. Individual failures include inattention to detail, lapses of memory, negligence, forgetfulness and carelessness. However, remedial action, which often suits a hierarchical management style, involves 98% concentration on individual failures and only 2% on organisational failures.

Systems failure

With most incidents being caused by organisational failures, OWAM favours the systems approach, with the right people in place to implement the processes and systems of care delivery. The systems approach takes a holistic view on the issue of failures and looks at complex organisations, where ill-defined responsibilities, policies and procedures and multifarious factors mean some degree of error is inevitable.

Organisations operating in hazardous circumstances have defences and safeguards in place to prevent risk being realised (see Figure 1 overleaf).

Professor Reason's 'Swiss cheese' model (see Figure 2 overleaf) tries to analyse near-misses and incidents which occur in healthcare settings by looking at the sequence of events which lead up to early detection or to an accident or incident.

This model can be used to look back at the conditions in which staff were working and the organisational context in which the incident or near-miss occurred. It shows that poor management decisions and organisational processes affect not only the local climate in which

Serious accidents don't just happen:

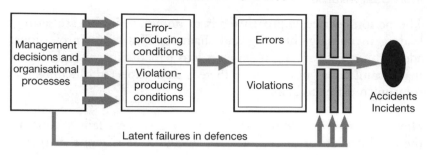

Figure 1: How accidents breach defences
Source: J Reason, 1994

clinical practice takes place, but also weaken the defences which could potentially prevent errors from becoming incidents.

Figure 2 is best understood if studied from right to left. Defences and safeguards may have holes that are continually opening, shutting, or shifting position. Usually hazards do not penetrate through all defences, but occasionally the holes will 'line up' because of active failures and latent conditions, enabling an incident to occur.

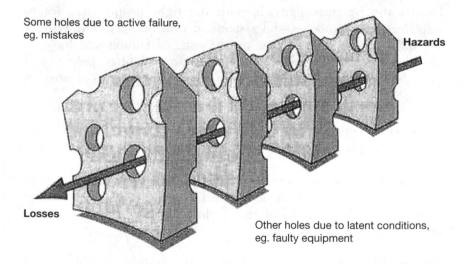

Figure 2: The Swiss cheese model of how defences, barriers, and safeguards may be penetrated by an accident trajectory.
Source: J Reason, 1997

Active failures

A key step in managing clinical risk is to identify active failures that can lead to immediate adverse consequences for patients.

These include:

- **staff memory lapses and mistakes** – through ignorance or mis-reading the situation

- **slips or failures** – such as picking up the wrong syringe or forgetting to carry out a procedure

- **violations** – deviations from safe practices, procedures or standards of care with no deliberate intention to do harm

There can also be deliberate departures from safe operating practices, procedures or standards – either due to deliberate errors or conflict with management.

Examples of active failures[6]

The significance of decelerations on a cardiotacograph (CTG) trace was not given sufficient weight, resulting in a prolonged labour and a brain-damaged baby.

A consultant overrode the decisions of the team without giving due consideration to their argument. He came in and took control of the situation without knowing the circumstances.

A patient's self-harm intentions were not taken seriously and were omitted from her care plan. The patient outlined her feelings of self-harm and these were discussed but not recorded or communicated to other staff groups.

Latent conditions

Latent conditions arise from fallible decisions, often taken by people not directly involved in the workplace. These factors may lie dormant in the workplace for long periods, before combining with other factors and active failures to penetrate or bypass defences.

They provide the conditions[5] under which unsafe acts occur, such as:

- high workload, time pressures, and fatigue

- inadequate knowledge, ability or experience
- inadequate supervision or instruction
- a stressful environment
- organisational change
- inadequate communication and documentation
- poor maintenance of equipment and buildings
- incompatible goals which can cause conflict

Latent conditions are always present but they can be identified and removed prior to causing an accident or incident. The culture and core beliefs of the organisation and the values of the staff need to change to deal with latent conditions on a proactive basis.

Examples of latent conditions[6]

There were no clear demarcation of roles and responsibilities and no agreed line of communication in a crisis.

There was general acceptance of faulty equipment being the norm, with a lax system for reporting faults. Staff felt there was no point in reporting faults when nothing happened as a result, and they felt that nobody wanted to know.

There was no system within the unit to ensure that lessons were learnt from serious incidents. They were just accepted as the norm and described as accidents waiting to happen.

System failures

Behind these error-producing conditions may lie a further set of wider organisational problems – known as system failures – which may be associated with a conflict between profit and safety, inadequate communication and deficient training. Examples include:

- incompatible goals between different staffing levels within the organisation
- no shared goals, commitment or vision throughout the organisation
- inadequate communication, with no clear strategy, information-sharing or two-way process to ensure involvement at all levels

- poor planning and scheduling leading to frustrations, delays and negative effects on patient care

- inadequate control and monitoring, with lack of leadership and failure to tackle issues, resulting in staff frustration and demotivation

- design failures stemming from a lack of consultation and involvement of users and patients

- deficient training with inadequate preparation and ongoing development to help staff cope with all eventualities

- inadequate maintenance management, with poor facilities and equipment

Avoiding adverse events

Analysis should focus on the organisational causes of near-misses and incidents, with much less focus on the individuals concerned. Adverse events,[7] near-misses and incidents can be avoided through:

- adequate communication

- meticulous, contemporaneous documentation

- adequate levels of supervision, responsibility and accountability

- up-to-date policies, procedures and guidelines

- safe, up-to-date clinical practice

- appropriate staffing and resources, and thus appropriate workload levels

- appropriate use of locums, bank and temporary staff

- safe organisational practices with adequate people management

- education and training for all staff

- safe systems of work

- performance management and staff appraisal systems

- healthy staff who are fit to practise

Tools of risk modification[8] are designed to promote proactive risk management, and help to provide a controlled environment of care in which the multidisciplinary team can minimise or eliminate the causes of identified risks. Having these safeguards in place will assist professionals in the audit and evaluation of their care delivery, with a feeling of local ownership and control.

Learning from mistakes

OWAM deals with how an ongoing analysis of near-misses and incidents can give the NHS rich detail on adverse outcomes and underlying causes. Awareness of the nature, causes and incidence of failures is a vital component of prevention – and prevention is cheaper than cure.

Lessons for the NHS from a serious adverse incident

Since 1985, at least 13 patients in the UK have died or been paralysed as a result of the accidental intrathecal (spinal) administration of a drug vincristine that is intended for intravenous administration only. This issue was highlighted in 2000 in OWAM. On 4 January 2001 a serious adverse incident of this type happened during the care of Wayne Jowett, an 18-year-old undergoing leukaemia treatment at Queen's Medical Centre in Nottingham. He subsequently died on 2 February 2001.

Systems failures

Two reports into the incident[7,9] highlight a variety of systems failures contributing to the incident. These range from operational practices – such as the pharmacy releasing drugs for intravenous and intrathecal use at the same time – to a lack of protocols for medical staff to follow when administering intrathecal chemotherapy. Training issues, such as a lack of induction for new specialist registrars on the ward, and communication issues – such as the consultant's expressed wish to see the patient when he arrived verbally rather than in the notes – all contributed to the incident. Labelling and packaging, and the fact that the syringe containing vincristine could be fitted to the intrathecal delivery system, were further contributing factors.

Action

The Department of Health pledged to reduce to zero, by the end of 2001, the number of patients dying or being paralysed by maladministered spinal injections. It has issued a circular,[10] outlining the action trusts should take. This includes: formal induction and appropriate training for all staff prescribing, dispensing or administering chemotherapy; a requirement for all intrathecal chemotherapy to be administered in a designated, separate area; and clear labelling of all drugs with life-threatening consequences.

It is possible to identify common themes or characteristics in failures, which should be of use in helping to predict and prevent further adverse events. Many healthcare incidents are preventable and all errors can be minimised. It is essential that lessons are learnt, and appropriate practices, policies and systems put in place to minimise recurrence.

Identifying clinical risk through claims

Analysing clinical negligence claims is one way of identifying common themes in adverse events in healthcare. However, within the UK we do not have a good database to learn from claims and to help establish good clinical risk modification programmes. This is due to the lack of central coordination and sharing of data, as highlighted in OWAM, but the situation should improve over time. A further restriction on learning from claims is that most adverse incidents do not result in a negligence claim.

Analysis of closed claims, available through firms of solicitors, law journals, the General Medical Council and some hospitals, highlights some common themes. The following 401 closed claims came from across the UK between March 1993 and July 1995. The analysis by specialty revealed the following:

UK experience

Obstetric	101	25.0%
Gynaecology	57	14.2%
Orthopaedics	49	12.2%
Anaesthetics	43	10.7%
Accident & emergency	30	7.5%
General surgery	28	7.0%
Other	93	23.4%
Total	**401**	**100%**

In a separate study in Scotland, data on 1,185 cases open at August 1995 revealed a similar pattern with slightly increased percentages in A&E and general surgery.

Scottish Office

Obstetrics & gynaecology	320	27%
Accident & emergency	202	17%
Orthopaedics	154	13%

General surgery	142	12%
Other	367	31%
Total	**1,185**	**100%**

Costs

The cost of litigation is continuing to rise in the UK and the costs associated with the 401 closed claims resulted in a total of £23,909,596 awarded, an average of £59,625 per case – excluding legal costs.

38% of the total costs of the awards went to obstetrics and gynaecology – obstetrics with £6,876,033 (28%) and gynaecology with £2,413,124 (10%). The average cost for obstetrics was £68,080 and for gynaecology, £42,335, again demonstrating that this is the most high-risk specialty.

Analysis by clinical specialty

A further analysis of the claims by specialty brought up a number of factors specific to each.

Obstetrics

Factors specific to this specialty include:

- Death or brain damage to the infant, due to birth asphyxia and inappropriate deliveries, are associated with a high proportion of claims.

- Inadequate foetal monitoring, including the recording of CTGs and pH levels of the foetus, leading to delay in treatments and intervention.

- Delays in performing caesarean sections due to a number of factors including inadequate training and supervision of junior medical staff. There may be an inadequately defined chain of command and a fear of upsetting teamworking. Staff may allow arguments to become personal instead of thinking of foetal and maternal well-being. There may be a lack of experienced personnel available to perform emergency surgery, and a lack of theatre facilities or staff.

- Delays in involving senior medical staff due to fears about appearing unable to cope, or the inappropriate attitude or responses of some senior staff.

- Intraoperative problems including equipment failures due to lack of maintenance, training in usage and regular checks. There may not always be back-up equipment if something malfunctions or is unsafe to use.

- Retained products such as placental tissue or swabs and negligent repairs of vaginal, third degree and episiotomy tears.

Gynaecology

Factors identified in gynaecology include:

- Damage to adjacent organs or vessels during surgery, and negligence during procedures.

- Failed communication, with a lack of explanation to the patient, which may contribute to an inadequate consent process.

- Sterilisation failures due to poor technique, or to inadequate explanation of the risks and benefits of the procedure and any alternatives.

- Retention of swabs, needles and products following surgery, without adequate surgical counts and checks on materials used during the procedure.

- Failure to diagnose, especially ectopic pregnancies and ovarian cysts, failure to undertake pregnancy testing prior to hysterectomies, and resultant complications.

Orthopaedics

Causes of successful litigation in orthopaedics include:

- Retained foreign bodies, diathermy burns and medical errors.

- Operative nerve damage and negligent performance of procedures.

- Broken or malfunctioning equipment such as drills and screws.

- Missed diagnoses, undiagnosed fractures or delays in diagnosis causing perceived worsening of condition.

- Inadequate consent and communication with the patient on the risks, alternatives and benefits of treatment, and in particular failure to warn the patient of potential complications.

- Post-operative complications such as infections, pressure sores and patient falls.

- Failure to train and supervise juniors appropriately.

Surgical specialties

Factors identified in surgery include:

- Technical errors, including the patient remaining aware of procedures when they are meant to be under general anaesthetic.

- Poor anaesthetic technique resulting in dental damage.

- Retained foreign bodies, including swabs, instruments, blades and needles.

- Diagnostic errors, such as misdiagnosed ectopic pregnancies and appendicitis.

- Post-operative complications may result when inadequate guidance is given to the patient.

Accident and emergency

In A&E, the factors identified were:

- Failures in diagnosis, many related to the interpretation of X-rays and inappropriate X-rays.

- Failures in training and supervision of junior doctors, with over 70% of claimants not being seen by a doctor more senior than a senior house officer. About 65% of incidents occurred when there were no middle or senior grade doctors present in the A&E department.

- Poor communication, lack of follow-up instructions, and negative attitudes.

Acting on analysis

Analysis of these claims helps to identify the areas where there is the potential for error, where lessons need to be learnt in order to change practice and behaviour, and where monitoring systems ought to be in place for early detection.

This allows for early identification, review and full investigation, and for action to be taken in order to prevent injuries and untoward

Common factors in claims

Factors common across all specialties and many of the 401 UK claims analysed included:

- inconsistent and poor record-keeping

- incomplete or missing documentation, especially the most crucial, such as CTG or investigation results that were claimed not to have been acted upon

- inability to locate the staff involved, with poor investigation at the time of the incident and no mechanism to track staff down

- poor information, communication and consent processes leading to patient dissatisfaction and anger

- unhelpful remarks and attitude problems

- inadequate care and attention

- poor explanation and no discharge information

outcomes to patients. Examples of good practice implemented as a result include the use of monitors to record the oxygen levels of patients during anaesthesia, and the identification of high-risk conditions presenting to an accident and emergency department which need to be assessed by senior doctors.

Learning from the US

In the US,[11] clinical risk modification programmes combine specialty-specific clinical guidelines, monthly reporting of clinical indicators, patient record review criteria and annual clinical practice surveys, in an effort to help providers focus on improving systems and practices that may expose patients to the risk of injuries. They are based on frequent analysis of their claims database, which helps to identify poor practice and areas for clinical improvement. In the UK and Europe we could learn some lessons from the approaches taken in the US, where risk management practices have been established for much longer.

Developments in clinical negligence

Avoiding health litigation has become an international priority. We now have increased public expectations and a more litigious society, with more people seeking compensation if they encounter an unexpected outcome or an adverse healthcare event.

Well-publicised cases, such as those of surgeon Rodney Ledward and the paediatric cardiac surgery service at Bristol Royal Infirmary (see KEY REFERENCES, piii) – plus the multiple murder conviction of former GP Harold Shipman – have given the Government and the healthcare professions a forceful push in the direction of quality improvement, accountability and care management. The result is a major impetus for change that is proceeding at a fast rate and is gaining momentum.

Clinical risk and litigation management strategies are on the national agenda, along with a number of other health quality initiatives, such as corporate and clinical governance, controls assurance, and patient empowerment.

The Woolf reforms to civil procedures

In the English legal system, the Woolf reforms to civil procedures were early products of this national recognition that high levels of clinical negligence litigation could no longer be tolerated. The clinical negligence pre-action protocol[12] arose from a review of civil litigation by the Lord Chief Justice, Lord Woolf, and subsequently the work of the Clinical Disputes Forum, a multidisciplinary group formed in 1997 as a result of the Woolf civil justice inquiry. The protocol is now part of a practice direction accompanying the civil procedure rules.

Commitment and steps

In the new system, parties to a clinical negligence dispute will be penalised by sanctions, including cost penalties, if they do not follow the protocol. The protocol covers two central areas, commitment and steps.

The commitment section gives guiding principles which healthcare providers, patients and their advisers are invited to subscribe to when dealing with patient dissatisfaction with treatment, and with complaints and potential claims.

The steps section sets out in a prescriptive form a recommended action sequence to be followed if litigation is a prospect. Issues covered include patients reporting any concerns and dissatisfactions to the healthcare provider where reasonably possible.

Healthcare providers should ensure that key staff, including claims and litigation managers, are appropriately trained and have some knowledge of healthcare law, complaints procedures, and civil litigation practices and procedures. Health service provider response times to key events such as record requests are stated.

Clinical negligence claims in the NHS (England)

- 23,000 claims were outstanding at 31 March 2000.

- 10,000 new claims were received and 9,600 claims settled in 1999–2000.

- Liabilities stood at £3.9 billion at 31 March 2000, up from £3.2 billion at 31 March 1999.

- Claims settled in 1999–2000 cost £386 million in England.

- In 65% of cases where settlements are up to £50,000, the costs of settlement are greater than the damages awarded.

- On average, claims settled in 1999–2000 had been on the books for five and a half years.

Source: National Audit Office 2001

Reform of the clinical negligence system

The 2001 National Audit Office report into clinical negligence[13] (see box) included an estimate for the first time of a £1.3 billion liability for incidents incurred but not reported. Up to 40,000 patients a year die as a result of hospital accidents, and one in 14 suffers an adverse healthcare event, such as diagnostic error or surgical mistake. Only a tiny proportion pursue any claim, but the number is on the increase.

As this book went to press, the Government was due to publish for consultation a white paper on the clinical negligence system, which includes proposals on ways to reduce the NHS litigation bill.

In the consultation document, entitled *Call for Ideas*,[14] the Chief Medical Officer (CMO) Professor Sir Liam Donaldson outlines several ways to speed up settlements for people injured by medical blunders or accidents in NHS hospitals or GP surgeries, including fixed-rate payments and no-fault compensation.

Comments are invited from NHS staff and patients. These will inform an expert panel led by the CMO, which will make recommendations early in 2002.

Changes under consideration

Options to be examined by the panel include a no-fault system, which could mean that NHS staff would not be blamed for problems. Some believe this would encourage doctors to be more open about their errors and improve their clinical practice, and discourage the practice of defensive medicine.

Other aspects of the system under consideration include structured settlements, which would see patients receiving periodic payments based on their future needs – such as nursing care – rather than a lump sum; fixed tariffs for specific injuries; and greater use of mediation rather than financial compensation.

The CMO is of the view that fundamental reform of clinical negligence is long overdue, as the current arrangements do not work for NHS staff or patients, and a faster and fairer system is needed. He says that a system where staff fear being dragged through the courts can lead to mistakes being covered up, at odds with government reforms to encourage more openness and learn from mistakes.

Curbing the compensation culture

It appears that the Government is concerned about the compensation culture growing in the NHS. Alan Milburn, the health secretary, is thought to favour fixed tariffs offered to victims along with non-financial compensation, such as regular nursing or other health services as necessary. The Government is keen to curb legal costs, and health department aides say the situation is worsening because of increased use of no-win, no-fee legal arrangements by people with minor claims.

Although patients will still be able to sue doctors, ministers are determined to ensure the new system is sufficiently generous that most will choose to avoid long legal proceedings. Milburn is also hoping that by lessening the chances of legal action he can create a more open culture among doctors and nurses that will enable potential errors to be identified before they happen, and procedures changed more easily in the wake of an incident to avoid a repetition.

NHS structures

Some NHS initiatives to improve the management of clinical risk, and thus improve outcomes and reduce claims, are already under way. The NHS Litigation Authority (NHSLA) was set up under section 11 of the *NHS Act 1977* and manages a number of schemes to control clinical risk, personal injury, property and other healthcare risks.

One of these schemes is the Clinical Negligence Scheme for Trusts (CNST) (see below) which helps NHS trusts pool the costs of liabilities arising from their clinical activities.

The NHSLA in April 1998 appointed a panel of 18 defence solicitors to handle litigation claims brought against NHS trusts. Previously the NHSLA had to work with nearly 100 defence firms. The rationale for the reduction was to enable the NHLSA to manage defence litigation practices more effectively by having a smaller number of firms. Quality of advice and service were also motivating factors. The panel was further reviewed in 2000 and the number of firms now stands at 15.

The Clinical Negligence Scheme for Trusts

The CNST[15] is a mutual pooling, pay-as-you-go arrangement for NHS trusts in England, designed to assist trusts in meeting the costs of clinical negligence claims. Similar schemes have been set up in Wales (Welsh Risk Pool), Scotland (Clinical Negligence and Other Risk Indemnity Scheme) and in the Republic of Ireland (Enterprise Liability Scheme). These schemes are aimed at promoting more effective risk, quality and claims management, resulting in better standards of patient care.

The CNST was launched in 1995 with voluntary membership. Its primary purpose was to give greater certainty to budgeting and planning by providing financial assistance to trusts in the event of a very large claim, a run of high claims or a serial claim, any of which could otherwise cause severe financial problems.

Trusts could choose to have different excess levels depending on their specialties, revenue, claims management and history. A discount of 5% in the first year was awarded on the basis of a completed self-assessment questionnaire, and evidence from supporting documentation of progress in implementing clinical risk management standards. Discount levels have been set for meeting compliance with the three levels of clinical risk standards.

Changes to CNST

As from 1 April 2002, substantial changes to the CNST are taking place following a review of its operation by the Department of Health and the NHSLA. Responsibility for managing clinical negligence claims and accounting for clinical negligence liabilities under the CNST will transfer from NHS trusts and primary care trusts to the NHSLA. The CNST will apply to all trusts and primary care trusts in England.

Benefits

The NHSLA says the benefits resulting from this change will be:

- increased financial incentive for risk management
- standardisation and benefits of scale in claims handling
- simpler and transparent accounting for clinical negligence
- better control of clinical negligence costs nationally
- easier financial management at health authority and trust level

Legal liability for clinical negligence will remain with the responsible body, but the NHSLA will manage all clinical negligence claims and account for all clinical negligence liabilities. Trusts will thus only account for contributions to the CNST and there will be no excess on claims. The NHSLA will instruct and negotiate with solicitors on all claims and will settle claims directly with claimants. However, it says trust staff currently employed in claims management will continue to undertake claims processing, liaison with management and clinicians, gathering witness statements and collating clinical records, as well as managing the interface with risk management.

The NHSLA says these changes should enable trusts to concentrate on prevention of negligence through risk management, and that the CNST in its new form will still provide a financial incentive for good risk management through contribution discounts. Discounts will still be based on an assessment of the trust's risk management activities against specified standards.

CNST standards

The CNST risk management standards were launched in April 1996 and updated in spring 2000. Eleven original standards have now increased to 14. Three of the original 11 have been revised, and there are three new standards. Standard 4 (incident reporting) and standard 9 (induction and training) have both been revised and have additional features. The former standard 11 (maternity care) has been renumbered as standard 12 and also has additional features. The new standards are standard 11 (clinical care), standard 13 (mental health and learning disabilities), and standard 14 (ambulance service). From 2001 an infection control standard has been added and a formal assessment against the criteria will commence in April 2002.

Standard 4: incident reporting

There are two additional features in standard 4. The first criterion, recommended by the General Medical Council (GMC), states: "In the interests of patient safety, openness and constructive criticism of clinical care is actively encouraged." The second additional criterion states: "The trust has a policy on the relationship between incident reporting and disciplinary action." According to the standard: "In order to encourage incident reporting, it is important that staff know where they stand with regard to disciplinary action if they report an incident where they are or may have been at fault. Any policy should treat all staff equally."

Standard 9: induction and training

Standard 9 is a revised standard with a number of additional features. The objective of the standard is to ensure that there are management systems in place to ensure the competence and appropriate training of all clinical staff. There are a number of criteria for this standard, many recommended by the GMC, including that:

- The trust has clear policies to ensure the health and well-being of clinical staff.

- There is a procedure to verify the registration of clinical staff.

- The trust has an induction system covering all temporary (locum, bank or agency) clinical staff to ensure that such employees are competent to perform the duties of their post.

- The trust has a clear policy requiring a consultant to have attended a relevant training programme before embarking upon techniques which are new to them, and which are not part of a research programme approved by the local ethics committee.

- Any person operating diagnostic or therapeutic equipment has a sufficient understanding of its use to do so in a safe and effective manner.

Standard 11: clinical care

Standard 11 is a new standard that is designed to ensure that "there are clear procedures for the management of general clinical care". There are a number of criteria for this standard, including that:

- The trust applies the advice of national confidential enquiries.

- There are specific clinical standards for each specialty.

- The trust can demonstrate that there is a clear documented system for management and communication throughout all stages of patient care.

- All specialties have in place an integrated policy that identifies and addresses the needs of the patient prior to, and in preparation for, discharge from the hospital.

- High-risk clinical areas are appropriately staffed at all times.

- Emergency surgery out of hours is reduced to a minimum.

- There are clear lines of accountability and responsibility for staff working in another organisation's facility.

Standard 12: maternity care

This standard has been renumbered and has some additional features and amendments, including:

- All midwifery and medical staff on labour wards should receive ongoing training in the use and interpretation of CTG recordings.

- There are clear arrangements regarding which professional is responsible for the patient's care at all times.

- There are detailed multidisciplinary policies for the management of all key conditions and situations on the labour ward, and these are subject to review at specified intervals.

- There is a named person with designated responsibility for maternity or labour ward matters.

- Emergency caesarean section can be undertaken rapidly and within a short enough period to eliminate unacceptable delay.

From April 2002 there will be a new enhanced maternity care standard. This will form a separate assessment for trusts providing maternity services and will address the links with the rest of the trust.

Standard 13: mental health and learning disabilities

This is a new standard relating to the management of care in trusts providing mental health and learning disability services. There are two basic criteria: first, that all service users are assessed for the possibility of self-harm or harm to others, and appropriate control measures are in place; second, that there is a multidisciplinary care programme approach.

Standard 14: ambulance service

Standard 14 is another completely new standard, designed to ensure that there are clear procedures for the management of clinical risk in trusts providing ambulance services.

There are four main criteria:

- Records are made of patients who refuse to travel or refuse treatment.

- Appropriate controls govern the use of medicines by paramedic staff.

- Patients suffering trauma or accident are transported to an institution appropriate to their clinical needs.

- There is clear decision-making regarding discontinuance of resuscitation attempts.

CNST levels

The CNST standards are aimed at ensuring that risk management is conducted in a focused and effective fashion, which is intended to have a positive contribution towards the improvement of patient care within member trusts. The standards have been set on three levels to encourage progression over time.

Level 1 focuses on the strategic issues and effectiveness of policies, procedures and strategies. Levels 2 and 3 focus on operational implementation, integration and cultural awareness of striving for continuous quality improvements. Each level must be achieved prior to being assessed at the next level, and only one assessment of a trust can be made in any one year. Each standard has a number of key features that are scored and weighted according to their relevant importance to effective risk management.

Assessing claims

Claims assessment standards, procedures and guidelines have been drawn up by the CNST to ensure that payments made to claimants are justified, appropriate, and equitable to other CNST members in terms of good claims handling and management. The overall aim is to ensure that genuine claimants receive an appropriate settlement. The CNST also suggests that trusts should carry out regular internal audit to ensure they meet the specified minimum standards within their claims handling procedures.

In time the CNST should have an extensive database on risk and claims management and be able to identify significant trends in litigation. This will provide powerful information that can be used proactively to manage clinical risk, and further clinical effectiveness initiatives – including benchmarking by clinical indicators, the production of appropriate guidelines as part of care pathways, and education and training programmes. The full CNST standards are available on *www.doh.gov.uk/riskman.htm*.

Impact of the CNST

Figures from 2000 show that more than seven out of 10 members of the CNST have now achieved compliance at level 1 of the risk management standards. However, only 7% have achieved level 2 and there is only one trust at level 3.

The number of trusts that have demonstrated compliance has risen steadily since the scheme was initiated – despite a slight dip between 1996 and 1997, when trusts first had to undergo an external assessment rather than performing self-assessment.

However, at least 23% of trusts have not yet achieved compliance at level 1; in some cases trusts' performance has slipped between assessment visits, some have lost level 1 and others have had to be reassessed because of trust mergers.

Areas requiring attention

The problem areas identified by the CNST as requiring attention are:

- Risk management strategies have been allowed to become out of date, or are inaccurate and have no ongoing review and evaluation.

- Clinical near-miss and incident reporting levels remain disappointing, with evidence that near-misses and incidents are either not being reported, or that there is inadequate feedback on incidents to staff.

- Documentary evidence to support alternative approaches to obtaining consent, and evidence of information given to patients, are not always available.

- The unified patient record is proving difficult to achieve in some trusts – particularly in multidisciplinary trusts, or trusts which have recently merged.

- Trusts need to improve induction training for new staff, particularly for doctors in the training grades, and for consultants.

Effecting change in clinical practice

In order to further evidence-based clinical risk management within healthcare organisations, there is a need to look at compliance with clinical guidelines and sharing best practice.

Finding the root cause

Root cause analysis involves the following steps

- outline sequence of events
- find and record each pertinent event
- avoid early judgment, blame or attribution
- concentrate on the facts
- look at why the incident occurred – causation
- look at how the incident occurred – system faults, active errors, latent failures, flawed defences
- situational factors – distractions, circumstances, triggers for latent failures

---

One way of starting to do this is by early recognition of near-misses and adverse healthcare events, and undertaking root cause analysis (see box overleaf) in order to identify areas of poor compliance, system failure, violation of procedures and the need for changes in clinical practice. It is only when this analysis is undertaken that lessons will be learnt and practice changed appropriately, as discussed in chapter 3.

Analysis of medication errors

In undertaking an analysis of medication errors, Figure 3 opposite shows the root causes of mistakes in the administration of drugs in a particular healthcare setting. This shows that education and training are factors in 60% of errors while distraction is a factor in only a minority of errors. Further analysis across a healthcare community revealed the areas where the drug errors were taking place. It found that 56% of all the errors surveyed occurred in the outpatient setting. Of these,

- 38% occurred in hospital outpatient clinics

- 25% in health centres or GP surgeries

- 7% in accident and emergency departments

- 7% in pharmacy

- 7% in day surgery units

- 16% in other outpatient settings

The survey added that the remainder of all errors surveyed (44%) occurred in the inpatient setting. Of these,

- 54% occurred in ward areas

- 16% in operating theatres

- 14% in ICU

- 16% in other inpatient settings

Breast cancer care case study

Another case study shows what can be revealed through root cause analysis, using a risk management information system.[16] The case examined was compliance with breast cancer clinical guidelines and an algorithm for agreed treatment patterns. The analysis resulted in the tightening up of guidelines, resulting in a reduction in claims and improved practice.

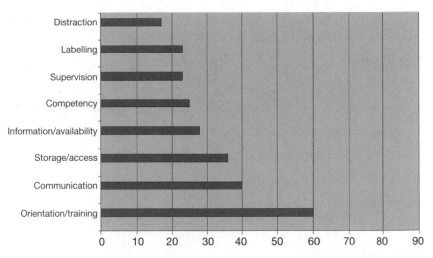

Figure 3: Root causes of medication errors

Root cause analysis and examples of common findings

Root cause analysis helps us to think about where to focus scarce resources, by considering the nature of adverse incidents, their severity and their frequency. Identifying why they happen, the risk management issues involved and how they can be prevented means that practice changes can be implemented through discussion with staff involved.

Where events occur – examples

Clinical risk management issues

- clinical judgment
- clinical decision-making process
- clinical systems
- patient follow-up

Coordination of care

- documentation
- results not in medical records

Communication issues

- lack of follow-through across areas
- discharge instructions
- integrated care management – guidelines not followed

Assessing compliance with the breast cancer algorithm and clinical guideline involved addressing the following factors:

- trends
- severity
- settings
- risk management issues
- root cause analysis and system failures
- clinical changes resulting
- experience – lessons to be learnt

Trends and severity

Breast cancer claims numbers are increasing, with an average cost of £400,000. Severity is high, with 55% of claims successful.

Impact on specialties

As Figure 4 opposite shows, claims associated with breast cancer cases may be made to a range of specialties – the most frequent being general medicine, followed by general surgery, obstetrics and gynaecology, radiology or imaging, pathology and accident and emergency.

A profile of the women and their condition found that the majority of them were under 49 years old. A total of 13% had a family history of breast cancer, 48% had discovered a breast lump and 14% presented with another breast complaint such as discharge, nodularity, dermatitis, thickening or pain.

Root cause analysis

Although the women were cared for in a number of different specialties, many common issues were found across the sectors of care. In 33% of cases, the clinician relied on a negative mammogram as evidence that a breast lump was not malign. In 19% of cases the mammogram was misread, and in a further 24% there was a low index of suspicion for breast cancer. Other factors accounted for the remaining 24%. As shown in Figure 5 opposite, clinical judgment was the largest risk management issue identified, with clinical systems second, followed by information-related risk issues, documentation, and communication.

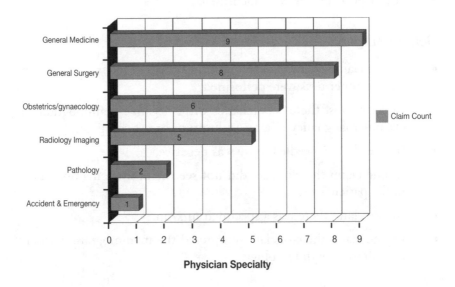

Figure 4: Specialty breakdown of breast cancer litigation

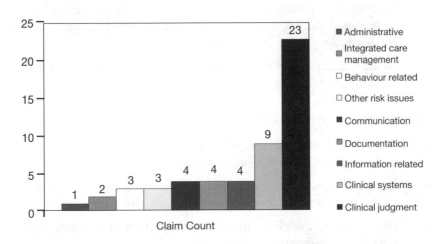

Figure 5: Risk management issues identified

When analysed by specialty, the following factors in clinical judgment and other aspects of care were identified:

General surgery

- In five claims, clinical examination gave a low index of suspicion and no other tests were performed.

- In six claims, there was reliance on a negative mammogram to exclude malignancy in a breast lump or breast complaint.

- In one claim a needle biopsy was negative.

- In one claim the clinician did not see the positive mammogram in the patient's record.

- In one claim there was a specimen mix-up.

- In one claim the clinician interpreted the mammogram without consultation with radiology.

Medicine

- In three claims, there was reliance on a negative mammogram to exclude malignancy in a breast lump.

- In two claims, breast examination was not performed or performed improperly.

- In one claim, a mammogram was not ordered because the lumps were noted during a patient's menstrual period. There was no further follow-up or breast examination.

- In one claim, there was a delay in follow-up of an abnormal mammogram.

Obstetrics and gynaecology

- In three claims, there was reliance on a negative mammogram to exclude malignancy in a breast lump.

- In two claims, there was clinical examination but no additional tests – one patient noted nodular changes, the other thickening.

- In one claim the clinician misinterpreted an addendum to the patient's mammogram report.

- In one claim, a breast lesion was aspirated but no fluid obtained. No additional tests were performed – the patient was pregnant, and told to return after her baby's birth.

- In one claim, a repeat needle aspiration specimen was not sent to the laboratory for analysis.

- In one claim, there was no follow-up of an abnormal mammogram

Highlights of the new algorithm

As a result of this analysis, changes have now been made to the algorithm used by clinicians. A screening mammogram enables patients to be put into different categories – for example, those in categories 4 and 5 (higher risk) will get an image-guided core biopsy of their breast lump, while those in categories 0–3 (lower risk) will get follow-up imaging in six months. Where there is a palpable mass on examination and the patient is less than 35 years old, ultrasound imaging will be performed.

Achieving risk modification

Risk management can be deployed in individual healthcare settings, and achieve risk modification, through:

- **Awareness and evaluation:** an in-depth assessment of the organisation's services and practices, and costs related to each, can begin to provide data from which potential risk areas can be identified. Included in this identification process are clinical and non-clinical components that contribute to the overall episode of care. Awareness is the first phase of risk modification.

- **Education and implementation:** the development of processes and interventions that begin to change undesirable practices or systems is the second phase of risk modification. This combines specific structural and procedural changes with an educational process.

- **Integration and support:** once changes and interventions are decided upon, a system for monitoring their integration into the organisation is needed to determine if the change has actually reduced the identified risk. Data collection, analysis, measurement, monitoring and re-evaluation form the third part of risk modification.

The risk modification process

This process can be shown as a flow of activity (see Figure 6) that fosters continuous risk modification and quality improvements in the system of healthcare delivery. This should be reflected within the organisation's risk management strategy.

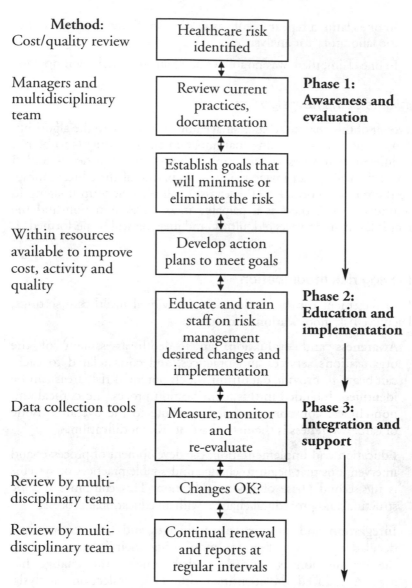

Method:		
Cost/quality review	Healthcare risk identified	
Managers and multidisciplinary team	Review current practices, documentation	**Phase 1: Awareness and evaluation**
	Establish goals that will minimise or eliminate the risk	
Within resources available to improve cost, activity and quality	Develop action plans to meet goals	
	Educate and train staff on risk management desired changes and implementation	**Phase 2: Education and implementation**
Data collection tools	Measure, monitor and re-evaluate	**Phase 3: Integration and support**
Review by multi-disciplinary team	Changes OK?	
Review by multi-disciplinary team	Continual renewal and reports at regular intervals	

Figure 6: Continuous risk modification and quality improvement in healthcare

Providing ongoing learning and improvements

Reports such as OWAM and *Building a Safer NHS for Patients* (see KEY REFERENCES, piii) highlight changes that all NHS organisations can start to implement – and many already have. Taking a holistic view of failure within organisations, and focusing on error management and error prevention, are important for developing organisations that can provide ongoing learning and improvements in quality and safety.

The NHS must use an active learning approach to help develop an informed culture where safety is an important feature. This also creates an environment in which people can learn from and respond to failures. Everyone knows that changing the culture of the organisation is hard work, but it is possible.

Developing an informed culture

Some of the actions to develop an informed culture will already have been undertaken by many organisations and include:

- raising the awareness of the costs of not taking risk seriously
- high priority given to reporting and feedback to staff, with action taken to prevent recurrence
- recognition of staff failure to identify serious events due to lack of awareness and training
- correction of weak systems and processes
- focusing on near-misses as well as incidents
- ensuring that concerns can be reported without fear, threats of disciplinary and punitive actions
- using external input to stimulate learning
- giving a high profile lead on the issues and demonstrating commitment of the trust board and senior medical and nursing clinicians

Learning from incidents

Learning from near-misses and incidents must take place on three levels. At the first level, individuals and the organisation involved in the particular incident can each draw their own lessons from it. More general lessons can be drawn from an analysis of the factors surrounding the incident. Finally, some learning can take place simply as a result of being made aware that a particular event has taken place. Learning lessons from near-misses and incidents is a key component of clinical governance and will be an essential part of delivering an organisational quality strategy.

A preventative focus

A preventative focus means looking at the conditions and systems of work. Each organisation needs to use appropriate tools to analyse their own safety performance, and recognise the background conditions that predispose to risky and unsafe practice. These can be monitored to assess the health of the organisation. A proactive approach is an essential component of any risk and quality management system, and must be embedded within the organisation.

References

See also KEY REFERENCES, piii

1. Wilson, JH (1998), 'Incident reporting', *British Journal of Nursing*, vol 7 no 11, pp 670–671.

2. Wilson, JH (1997), 'The Clinical Negligence Scheme for Trusts', *British Journal of Nursing*, 1997, vol 6, no 20.

3. Toft, B (1992), 'The failure of hindsight', *Disaster Prevention and Management*, vol 1, no 3.

4. Reason, J (1997), *Managing the Risk of Organisational Accidents*, Ashgate, Aldershot.

5. Overveit, J (1998), *Health Service Quality*, Brunel University, London.

6. Vincent, C, Taylor-Adams S, Stanhope N (1998), 'A framework for analysing risk and safety in clinical medicine', *BMJ* vol 316: pp1154–7.

7. Toft, B (2001), *External inquiry into the adverse incident that occurred at Queen's Medical Centre, Nottingham, 4 January 2001*, DoH, London. (*www.doh.gov.uk/qmcinquiry*)

8. Wilson, JH, Tingle, JH (1999), *Clinical risk modification: a route to clinical governance*, Butterworth Heinemann, Oxford 1999.

9. Woods, K (2001), *The prevention of intrathecal medication errors*, DoH, London. (*www.doh.gov.uk/imeprevent*)

10. Health Service Circular 2001/022, *National guidance on the safe administration of intrathecal chemotherapy*.

11. MMI Companies, Inc (1994), *Clinical Risk Modification Programs*, Deerfield, Illinois, USA.

12. Tingle, JH, Cribb, A (1995), *Nursing, Law and Ethics*, Blackwell Publishers, London.

13. National Audit Office (2001), *Handling Clinical Negligence Claims in England*, The Stationery Office, London.

14. Department of Health (2001), *Clinical negligence: what are the issues and options for reform?*, a "call for ideas".

15. Clinical Negligence Scheme for Trusts (2000), *Risk Management Standards and Procedures Manual of Guidance*, Willis, Bristol.

16. Risk Management Foundation and Marsh (2001), *Executive Information Systems for Root Cause Analysis*, Harvard Medical Group, Boston, USA.

Further information

The full CNST standards are available at *www.doh.gov.uk/riskman.htm.*

5 Clinical governance

Jo Wilson

This chapter covers:

- **The concept of clinical governance**

- **Dimensions of clinical governance**

- **The role of the National Institute of Clinical Excellence**

- **The role of the Commission for Health Improvement**

- **National service frameworks and performance assessment**

- **The NHS Plan and subsequent changes**

- **Clinical audit**

Clinical governance in healthcare is concerned with the consistent improvement in the quality of clinical care across whole organisations. It encompasses all the processes needed to achieve the highest quality clinical practice possible, within available resources.

It should provide a means of developing routines, so that looking at quality of care and identifying risks becomes an everyday part of life in healthcare delivery. Clinical governance presents a major opportunity for health professionals as it gives them the authority they need to make health service provision work more effectively.

Variations in both quality of care and its delivery suggest that many of the principles which should underpin any quality service are not always addressed. The reasons for this are complex, and may relate to:

- a narrow focus in the training of healthcare professionals

- boundaries and barriers between professional groups

- an inability to accept the need for and implement change

- fear of failure, blame and threats to clinical autonomy

- a poor record in effective teamworking

The concept of clinical governance ensures that quality of care is central to the delivery of care for all professional groups. It aims to ensure clear systems are in place to encourage healthcare professionals to work towards quality standards and check that they are doing so.

Clinical governance in the NHS

Systems of clinical governance outlined in the white paper *The New NHS: Modern, Dependable* (see KEY REFERENCES, piii) mark a fundamental and significant shift towards involving clinicians in quality, security and accountability in healthcare delivery. The paper states: "The Government will require every NHS trust to embrace the concept of clinical governance, so that quality is at the core, both of their responsibilities as organisations, and of each of their staff as individual professionals." Legislation following this white paper has imposed new duties on NHS trusts of quality of care and partnership working.

In *A First Class Service: Quality in the NHS* (see KEY REFERENCES, piii) clinical governance is defined as "a framework through which the NHS organisations are accountable for continuously improving the quality of their services, and safeguarding high standards of care by creating an environment in which excellence in clinical care will flourish". The principles of clinical governance apply to all those who provide or manage patient care services in the NHS.

Principles of clinical governance

Clinical governance incorporates a number of processes. These include:

- clinical audit

- the use of evidence-based practice

- promoting clinical effectiveness

- detecting and investigating adverse healthcare events

- analysing the root causes of adverse events

- improving practice as a result of complaints, analysis of adverse events, and monitoring standards and outcomes of care

These processes can be enhanced by the use of good quality clinical data, so that poor clinical practice can be recognised early and dealt with. Good practice should be systematically disseminated both within and outside the organisation and clinical risk reduction programmes of a high standard should be in place. Clinical governance has placed a duty of responsibility on all healthcare professionals to ensure that care is satisfactory, consistent and responsive.

Audit programmes and confidential enquiries

There is an expectation for all clinicians to fully participate in audit programmes, including specialty and subspecialty national external audit programmes, and the four confidential enquiries which now come under the responsibility of the National Institute for Clinical Excellence (NICE). These cover:

- maternal deaths
- stillbirths and deaths in infancy
- perioperative deaths
- suicide and homicide by people with mental illness

Clinical governance checklist

Healthcare organisations which are in step with clinical governance display some or all of the following attributes.

- Clinical quality improvements at ground level are integrated with an overall quality improvement programme.

- Good practice is systematically disseminated.

- Clinical risk reduction programmes using action plans and risk registers are in place.

- Evidence-based practice systems are in place.

- Adverse healthcare events and near-misses are detected and openly investigated; their root causes are analysed and lessons are learnt.

- Complaints are dealt with positively and the information is used to improve the organisation and its care delivery.

- High-quality data is used to monitor clinical care and support professionals in delivering quality care.

- Clinicians are encouraged to develop clinical leadership skills and manage performance, as part of self-regulation and assessment.

- Clinicians embrace continuing professional development.

- Staff are supported in their duty to report concerns about colleagues' professional conduct, and early action is taken to support the individual and remedy the situation.

- Poor clinical performance is dealt with appropriately to minimise harm to patients and other staff.

Dimensions of clinical governance

There are three dimensions to clinical governance which are:

- **Corporate accountability** for clinical performance, with the chief executive or the chair of the governing body taking overall responsibility, and a board subcommittee led by a clinician such as the medical director or chief nurse. There should be clear lines of leadership, responsibility and accountability for the overall quality of clinical care, stakeholder involvement and performance management.

- **Internal mechanisms** for improving clinical performance and delivering quality, including individual accountability, and professional self-regulation. Professional self-regulation gives health professionals the ability to set their own standards of professional practice, conduct and discipline. Staff looking after patients must be competent, up to date, properly trained and supervised. They must respond quickly to patients if things go wrong, and learn from healthcare mistakes. There should be an emphasis on lifetime learning through continuing professional development, as an integral part of quality improvement. Staff should be involved in shaping the healthcare delivery system and planning improvements to patient care.

- **External mechanisms**, such as review by the Commission for Health Improvement (CHI).[1] This is a statutory body responsible for reviewing the NHS, to support those who are developing and monitoring clinical quality. CHI provides national leadership on clinical governance and, through a rolling programme of local reviews, ensures that service providers have local systems to monitor, assure and improve clinical quality.

CHI also has the capacity to offer specific support on request when local organisations face particular clinical problems, and to conduct investigations to identify the sources of particular problems and help organisations find lasting remedies. CHI will assess NHS progress in achieving the standards set in the national service frameworks (NSFs), and uptake of NICE guidance, and will oversee critical incident enquiries to ensure the best outcomes for patients and the service. CHI will be discussed in more detail later in the chapter.

These three dimensions help to ensure there are proper processes in place for continually monitoring and improving clinical quality. Quality is monitored not only by CHI, but also by the national performance framework, the national survey of patient and user experience and the trust board. Figure 1 shows the Department of Health's representation of the clinical governance standard-setting, implementation and monitoring process.

Key elements of clinical governance

Clinical governance provides a framework through which clinicians and managers recognise their individual and collective responsibilities and accountabilities for care quality, and by which the healthcare organisation fulfils its statutory duty of quality of care.

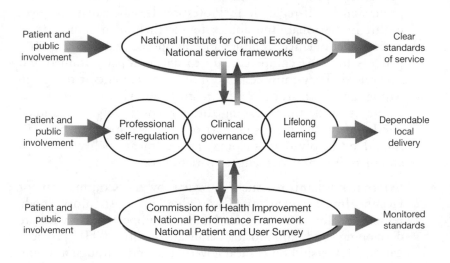

Figure 1: The DoH view of the clinical governance process

Most of the elements of clinical governance are not new to good clinicians and managers, but the framework provided by clinical governance brings them together. It thus provides a protective mechanism for both public and staff, who know that their local healthcare organisations are actively developing structures to improve quality and standards of patient care. Figure 2 demonstrates this.

1. Patient
2. Clinical Effectiveness
3. Continuous Quality Improvement
4. Clinical/Social Governance

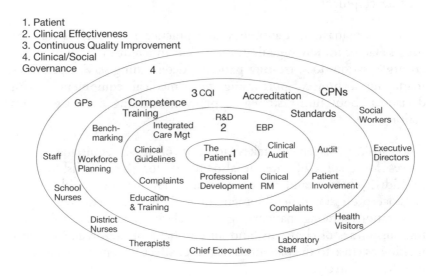

Figure 2: The components required for clinical governance

The elements of clinical governance which will be discussed here include:

- risk management – including addressing clinical risk and risk modification

- corporate governance, which in the NHS is implemented through controls assurance

- best practice and appropriate care

- the standards set by NICE and national service frameworks

- the monitoring role of CHI and performance assessment

- lifelong learning, professional self-regulation and clinical audit

Risk management

Risk management can be regarded as the lynch-pin connecting all the elements of clinical governance, and connecting clinical governance and controls assurance. The clinical governance framework encompasses all aspects of high-quality provision, such as quality assurance strategies, continuous quality improvements, clinical effectiveness, clinical audit, risk management and organisational and staff development.

Good risk management awareness and practice at all levels is a critical success factor for any organisation. Risk is inherent in everything that an organisation does: treating patients, determining service priorities, managing a project, purchasing new medical equipment, taking decisions about future strategies, or even deciding not to take any action at all.

Good risk management takes account of legal requirements and strives for quality of care. It also allows for the establishment of multidisciplinary standards of care and best practice guidelines to enhance professional development of nursing and medicine. Higher expectations among patients, greater clarity about the roles and responsibilities of clinicians, and an emphasis on devolving decision-making as close to the patient as possible, affect the entire spectrum of healthcare delivery.

Managing cost and quality of care

Most senior managers, nurses and doctors find that the environment in which they operate has grown turbulent and complex with increasing demands on resources and increases in workload. They must monitor patient activity and evaluate services through clinical audit – while controlling costs and providing accessible and equitable services with relevance to the local population's healthcare needs. The gatekeepers of healthcare, on behalf of their clients, must look for the best and most efficient healthcare delivery systems, giving the best value for money.

To improve value, providers must understand and use the link between its two basic components – cost and quality. Both the cost and quality of care are components in determining the value of the healthcare delivered, and both are elements of healthcare risk. Managing these elements of risk may be termed healthcare risk modification. The focus of healthcare risk modification is on the systems and practices that affect patient care, in order to manage the overall cost and appropriateness of care delivered.

Clinical risk and risk modification

Clinical risk management (see chapter 4 for a more in-depth look at clinical risk) is the systematic identification, assessment and reduction of risks to patients and staff, through:

- providing appropriate, effective and efficient levels of patient care

- prevention and avoidance of adverse incidents and events

- learning lessons and changing behaviour as a result of near-misses, incidents and adverse outcomes

- communication and documentation of care in a comprehensive, objective, consistent and accurate way

Modification is the changing of circumstances, the environment and behaviour to lower the potential for and amount of healthcare risk. Risk management tools help to identify areas where continuous quality improvements can be made. The result is improved outcomes and patient satisfaction.

Communication

Poor communication between professionals and with patients is the commonest reason for patients or relatives to make complaints, or even pursue litigation in order to acquire the necessary explanations and information. The Medical Protection Society estimates that in 92% of cases presented to it over a three-year period, failure to communicate featured as a major component of the case. This is underpinned by poor record-keeping with over 78% of cases having poor documentation.

In addition, the charity Action for Victims of Medical Accidents estimates that more than 50% of the complaints it receives are linked to communication problems. In order to modify clinical risk and manage it appropriately, the two best forms of risk prevention are effective communication and excellent documentation.

Management should evaluate the effectiveness of clinical practice, patient satisfaction and outcomes and examine the frequency, severity and defensibility of claims. This does not mean practising defensive medicine but having the best defensibility in place if and when things do go wrong. Arriving at a broader interpretation of risk management presents us with risk solutions.

Corporate governance and controls assurance

Corporate governance is another way of addressing risk management in the NHS – one that stems from efforts to improve the way businesses are run.

Effective corporate governance requires all government departments to meet the principles outlined in what is known as the Combined Code – a statement of the principles of internal control which was originally developed for the London Stock Exchange in 1998. In 1999 this was followed by the Turnbull guidance on internal controls (see KEY REFERENCES, piii).

These principles require that an organisation has in place sound internal control systems for identifying risks relating to the achievement of aims and objectives, evaluating the nature and extent of those risks and of managing them effectively, efficiently and economically. Within the NHS, all organisations are required to sign an annual statement of internal control to provide assurance to patients, staff and other stakeholders that such a system is in place.

Controls assurance is a system of management that is fundamental to corporate and clinical governance in the NHS. It exists to inform NHS boards about significant risks within the organisation for which they are responsible. It is intended to assist NHS staff, including chief executives and board members, to identify risks, to help them determine unacceptable levels of risk, and to then decide on where best to direct limited resources to eliminate or reduce those risks.

One of the fundamental assumptions of controls assurance is that all statutory and mandatory requirements with which NHS organisations need to comply address a risk of some sort. In other words, these requirements exist because of an identified need to control a risk that could threaten the organisation, the people, or the environment. Similarly, best practice guidance exists to advise on accepted, although not always evidence-based, options for dealing with potential risks. Thus non-compliance with standards and risk are synonymous in the context of controls assurance.

Best clinical practice and appropriate care

Clinical governance is difficult to achieve if it is unclear what the standards of practice ought to be. In order to establish best clinical, and in time, evidence-based practice, healthcare practitioners should identify areas in their practice from which clear clinical questions can be formulated. This will be supported by identifying evidence available from the literature, critically appraising the evidence for validity and clinical usefulness, and then implementing and incorporating findings into practice. The loop must then be completed by ongoing measurement of performance against expected outcomes or against peer review.

Appropriateness of care must become a major focus of developing best clinical practice, quality and clinical governance. However, it is difficult to find a clear definition of appropriateness of care.

Defining 'appropriateness' of care

Appropriateness can be seen as the optimum point of balance between liability and quality – so you have defensibility in terms of processes and systems if things do go wrong, and also the quality assurance standards to demonstrate a controlled environment of care (see Figure 3). Clinical and cost effectiveness must be considered to ensure that

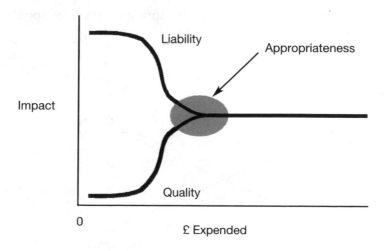

Figure 3: New definition of best clinical practice

scarce resources are used effectively, and not to practise defensive medicine for fear of litigation.

Preliminary data suggests (see Figure 4) that as quality increases in one direction to meet patients' perceived expectations and to combat fears of litigation, it reaches a meeting point with the appropriateness of treatment and beyond that point, appropriateness declines. Appropriate treatment is that which falls in line with evidence-based research and practice and clinical effectiveness.

Appropriateness must become the focus of quality when discussing whether interventions should be undertaken and whether they are in line with best practice. Best clinical practice based on research and evidence-based practice can help all trusts to demonstrate a controlled and high-quality environment of care based on patient requirements.

National Institute for Clinical Excellence (NICE)

The work of NICE is a key part of government efforts to define best practice and appropriate care and to provide clinical guidance at a national level. It has been created to promote clinical and cost effectiveness through clinical guidelines, best practice and audit.

The functions of NICE include:

* advising NHS professionals on the appropriate use of specific health technologies following technology appraisal

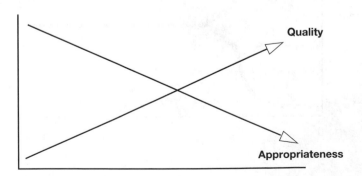

Figure 4: Quality and appropriateness

- advising NHS professionals on the appropriate management of specific conditions bearing both clinical and cost effectiveness in mind

- responsibility for service delivery guidelines for cancer

- advising health professionals of methodological advice on monitoring adherence to technology appraisal advice, and proposing audit criteria and methods

- commissioning and supporting national clinical audits conducted by national collaborating centres

- commissioning and supporting the national confidential enquiries and disseminating advice on reducing mortality and other serious adverse events

Along with NSFs, NICE is responsible for setting standards for service delivery, which are implemented at a local level and monitored by performance assessment and CHI (see Figure 1, p112).

Frameworks have been developed for cancer, mental health, older people and cardiology services. The National Priorities Guidance 2000/01–2002/03 cover the following areas:

- reducing waiting lists and times

- prompt and effective emergency care

- maintaining financial stability

- restoring working balances

- prevent and control communicable disease especially:

  - hospital-acquired infection

  - reduction in anti-microbial resistance

  - meeting immunisation targets

In Scotland, the Scottish Intercollegiate Guidelines Network (SIGN) regularly produces clinical guidelines. These, along with other sources of evidence, such as professional journals, guidelines from professional bodies and reviews such as the *Effective Healthcare Bulletin* produced by the University of York, help to underpin clinical governance efforts.

National service frameworks (NSFs)

NSFs are another strand of government efforts to provide better guidance to the NHS on what it ought to be doing. These go beyond a strictly clinical remit, in that they set both national clinical standards and define service models for specific services or care groups – including coronary heart disease, mental health and older people. The national cancer plan has set out standards for cancer care. Other NSFs for diabetes, children's services and renal care are under way.

NSFs do the following:

- set national standards and define service models for a specific service or care group

- lay out comprehensive programmes for improving care with annual targets, challenges and opportunities for healthcare providers

- put in place programmes to support implementation

- set out evidence-based standards, goals and milestones that primary healthcare teams, primary care groups and trusts must meet

- establish performance measures against which progress within an agreed timescale can be measured

Commission for Health Improvement (CHI)

Standard-setting at a national and local level lies at one end of the clinical governance spectrum; once efforts have been made to improve standards, assessment is needed. At a national level, assessment of progress against clinical standards is performed through CHI and the performance assessment framework.

The *Health Act 1999* requires CHI to review clinical governance arrangements in NHS organisations. CHI is a statutory body that provides independent scrutiny of local efforts to improve quality and to help address any serious problems.

It is conducting a rolling programme of external review for each NHS trust once every four years, to ensure that effective systems to continuously improve patient care are in place and that demonstrable improvement does take place. If a problem is identified regionally with a particular organisation prior to the planned programme, CHI will make an immediate visit to assess the situation.

Core functions of CHI

The core functions of CHI are to:

- support, develop and disseminate clinical governance principles
- independently scrutinise local governance arrangements to support, promote and deliver high-quality services
- advise on local clinical governance arrangements
- review the implementation of NSFs and NICE guidelines
- identify serious or persistent clinical problems
- concentrate on clinical issues and management issues where these are contributing to clinical problems
- increasingly take on responsibility for overseeing and assisting with external NHS incident inquiries in England and Wales as appropriate

The CHI review process

CHI has designed a review process that allows it, in any NHS organisation, to assess:

- who is accountable for the quality of patient care, and how the systems for accountability work
- the systems and processes for monitoring services
- the systems and processes for improving services

The CHI review process for acute hospitals lasts for 24 weeks and has four stages:

- collection of data and information from the hospital – including individual meetings with members of the public and other local organisations/patient groups and a staff survey
- a visit to the hospital by a trained team, which includes a nurse, a doctor, a manager, a lay person and a therapy professional
- the production of a written report of the assessment process
- formulation of an action plan by the hospital

The CHI review is fed back to the healthcare providers involved and a report is made public. The reports are firmly based on the patient experience. They will give a fair picture of the healthcare organisation, celebrating areas of good practice, but not shrinking from mention of areas that need attention.

CHI reports are freely available on the internet at *www.chi.nhs.uk*. They provide the information needed to develop and improve the services that each healthcare organisation offers to its patients.

National performance assessment

The NHS national framework for assessing performance judges how well each part of the NHS is doing to deliver quality services, although it is more concerned with organisational aspects of NHS service than with a purely clinical focus. The indicators focus on six areas which are:

- health improvement
- fair access to services
- effective delivery of appropriate healthcare
- efficiency
- patient and carer experience
- health outcomes of NHS care

Mature and responsible use of the information could support clinical governance, leading to improvements in quality of care where local investigation highlights any shortcomings.

DoH performance indicators

In September 2001 the Department of Health published the first performance ratings for acute NHS trusts, allocating them zero to three stars depending on performance against certain indicators. During 2001, all NHS organisations have also been expected to take part in local modernisation reviews, identifying what needs to be done in order to carry out the NHS Plan (see KEY REFERENCES, piii).

The Department of Health is consulting on performance indicators to be used in subsequent years, under a range of headings from coronary heart disease to hospital-acquired infection. It will continue to produce a set of performance indicators each year, and will work closely with CHI and the Audit Commission to maintain a consistent approach between performance indicators and the performance rating system.

The NHS Plan

The concept of clinical governance preceeds the NHS Plan (see KEY REFERENCES, piii), but much of the ambitious and far-reaching reform outlined in the plan, published in 2000, has a bearing on it. The plan promised:

- investment in NHS facilities and staff

- changes for patients, including greater choice and protection

- cutting patient waiting times, improving health and reducing inequality

- changes for NHS doctors, including new consultant contracts and new quality-based contracts for GPs

- new responsibilities and changes for NHS nurses, midwives, therapists and other NHS staff

- changed NHS systems

New bodies have appeared – such as the Modernisation Agency, whose stated aims are to "coordinate work to modernise services to meet the needs and convenience of patients" and to "coordinate management and leadership development to foster leadership talent at all levels within the health service".

The new organisational bodies will include:
- NHS Modernisation Agency
- National Independent Reconfiguration Panel
- National Performance Fund
- The NHS Leadership Centre
- NHS Appointments Commission
- National Clinical Assessment Authority
- NHSplus: National Agency
- Patient Advocacy and Liaison Service (Pals)

- UK Council of Health Regulators
- patients' forums
- Citizens Council (NICE)

Some of these new organisations and groups will inevitably have an impact on clinical risk and health litigation management policies and procedures. A new and more effective complaints system looks likely to be introduced, making it more independent and responsive to patients. Patients will have a firmer and an official platform from which to voice opinions and concerns. The initiatives will give patients more of a say in what happens, locally and nationally. Patients will have direct responsibility on every NHS trust board, elected by the patients' forum. The forum will be supported by the Patient Advocacy and Liaison Service (Pals) and will have the right to visit and inspect any aspect of the trust's care at any time. Pals' staff and forum members will also have access to the new NHS Leadership Centre's programmes.

Other reforms are also under way, such as reform to the way health professionals are regulated, and to the way that doctors' performance is assessed and managed – with help from the new UK Council of Health Regulators and the National Clinical Assessment Authority. Reforms to the complaints procedure have been proposed, and a review of the clinical negligence system is under way with a white paper due early in 2002.

Measures for greater patient involvement

To try and give patients greater involvement in healthcare, the following measures were announced in November 2001:

- Patient advice and liaison services are to be established in every NHS trust and primary care trust.

- A nationwide independent complaints advocacy service will be established to help patients pursue formal complaints through the NHS complaints procedure.

- A patients' forum in every trust will monitor and review the services provided by the trust and feed back local peoples' views.

- A new national body, the Commission for Patient and Public Involvement in Health, will coordinate patients' forums and local ICAS (Independent Complaints Advocacy Service).

The vision of the NHS Plan is to offer people fast and convenient care delivered to a consistently high standard. Services will be available when people require them, tailored to their individual needs. The NHS Plan is ambitious, radical and is based upon investment and reform, without which it will not be achievable. If these are not forthcoming, it will make the work of clinicians and managers harder because it has raised expectations of modernisation and rebuilding of NHS services.

Three aspects of quality

Delivering quality standards at a local level will very much depend on three elements:

- proper clinical governance

- the establishment and maintenance of lifelong learning

- ongoing professional self-regulation

Lifelong learning

Lifelong learning is an investment in quality that underpins clinical governance and it is important for the recruitment and retention of well-trained professionals. It also has to meet the needs of both health professionals and the NHS.

The NHS human resources strategy has addressed suggestions of how this will be achieved in order to provide the appropriately trained staff to give the best services and quality of care to patients. The NHS will be aiming to recruit and retain a quality workforce which has the capacity, skills, diversity and flexibility to meet the needs of the service. People management is covered in depth in chapter 9.

Professional self-regulation

Health and social care professionals set standards for professional practice, but usually on a uniprofessional basis. A move is beginning towards sharing best practice and working on a multidisciplinary basis through integrated care. This will help to ensure better professional self-regulation in the delivery of quality patient services, with professions being openly accountable for the standards and their enforcement.

Clinical audit has an important role in professional self-regulation. It enables clinicians to hold a mirror to their everyday work and, through discussion with peers and guidance from their professional bodies, make any relevant changes. For this very reason the professional bodies are increasingly requiring that clinical audit is a key component of all specialist training, and are encouraging them to continue such practice beyond their training.

Health commissioners and NHS trusts also need to encourage and support clinicians to include audit in their professional self-regulation and continuing educational development programmes. This includes ensuring that adequate resources, including protected time and support, are available. It also includes sharing the information and implications of clinical audit studies, which should be integrated into the clinical risk and clinical governance strategies to ensure that changes do occur, and that lessons are learned and shared throughout the healthcare system.

Clinical audit

Clinical audit is a crucial tool for securing improvements in the quality of patient care. One of the key components of clinical governance is that all clinicians should participate in internal and external clinical audit systems.

Clinical audit provides a comprehensive framework for quality improvement activity and processes for monitoring clinical care, using good information and clinical record systems.

Getting the basics right is essential. Clinical audit must be effective and good systems must not be allowed to deteriorate. It provides a formal approach to questioning clinical practice and developing new practices, and to ensuring these meet continuous quality improvements and clinical outcomes. It considers the effectiveness, efficiency and humanity of care and can be used to enhance education and develop clinical excellence by dealing with the structure, process and outcomes of healthcare.

Benefits of effective clinical audit

An effective clinical audit programme helps to give necessary reassurance to patients, clinicians and managers that an agreed quality of service is being provided within available resources. It can improve standards of care, raise awareness of costs, eliminate waste and inefficiency, and form a valuable educational tool for clinicians and their peers, juniors and other professionals. It is an educational process for clinicians, identifying inappropriate and inefficient clinical practices and inadequate support.

Clinical audit can lead to increased consumer awareness and choices about healthcare, as information becomes more readily available about clinical activity, quality of service and health outcomes. It has an important role in risk management, revealing where care is ineffective or below acceptable standards, and in encouraging more effective care and improved clinical outcomes.

Clinical audit and clinical governance

Clinical audit (see Figure 5), through the monitoring of standards and best practice, can assist clinicians in having robust processes to assess the effectiveness, efficiency and appropriateness of the clinical care they provide. This ties in with clinical governance when standards are not met or best practice is not being applied, and interventions are needed to fix the problem through internal scrutiny. This is supplemented by open and external review and participation in national audit programmes, including specialty and subspecialty national external audit programmes endorsed by CHI.

Clinical audit: monitoring standards and best practice

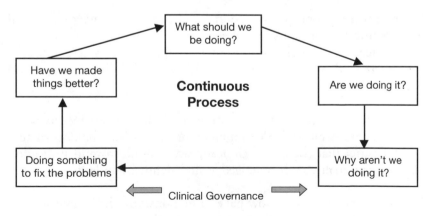

Figure 5: The clinical audit cycle

Clinical governance places a duty of responsibility on all healthcare professionals to ensure that care is satisfactory, consistent and responsive, with each individual responsible for the quality of their clinical practice as part of professional self-regulation. Clinical governance strengthens systems of quality assurance and clinical audit by promoting evaluation of clinical standards, better utilisation of evidence-based practice and learning lessons from poor performance. The clinical governance framework builds upon professional self-regulation and performance review; it takes account of existing systems of quality control and includes all activity and information for quality improvements.

Clinical and cost effectiveness

Clinical audit should be an activity that aims to produce change where change is necessary, and shares lessons to be learnt as well as working towards the delivery of services of the highest possible standard. However, the debate about clinical versus cost effectiveness and affordability must be considered.

A balance needs to be struck between effectiveness, appropriateness and acceptability. Inevitably, no healthcare activity can be perfect when judged against all these different criteria. A judgment will be required about what is reasonable. Resources will always be limited, and clinical audit should play a leading part in ensuring optimal use of resources.

Successful clinical governance

In order to fulfil both organisational and professional governance, all of the clinical professions must have structures and systems of clinical governance to maintain professional accountability. These must be integrated and reconciled with NHS accountability systems and structures at all levels.

The key to successful implementation of clinical governance is to be able to demonstrate the development of an accountability structure which ensures that changes in clinical practice result from identification of failures in quality and are judged against defined standards.

Healthcare organisations now have to demonstrate that they use clear lines of accountability, reporting mechanisms, risk management and ongoing quality measures to meet the governance agenda.

The role of clinical audit

Clinical audit is a vital part of clinical governance in that it focuses on the patient and the use of resources, the care given and the outcomes achieved. It provides systematic reviews of treatments, and the lessons learnt will improve standards, reduce clinical risk exposure and raise quality of care. Quality improvements cover three main areas: more flexible access to services; greater sensitivity to individual treatment needs; and improvements in technical competence.

Clinical audit also furthers clinical governance by enhancing lifelong learning through education and developing clinical excellence through the assessment processes, systems and outcomes of healthcare delivery. However, it must be remembered that clinical audit is a means to an end and not an end in itself: there must be ongoing re-evaluation for assurance of best and up-to-date practice.

Restoring public confidence

Clinical governance will have an important part to play in restoring public confidence in healthcare delivery through demonstrating quality assurance and control mechanisms. Patients and their families place trust in healthcare professionals and they need to be assured that their treatment is up to date, and effectively applied by staff whose skills have kept pace with evidence-based practice and new techniques.

Clinical governance must be seen as going hand in glove with clinical risk management in terms of modifying healthcare providers' behaviour to provide safe, effective and high-quality patient care. Quality and risk are two sides of the same coin and must work in synergy together to provide better patient care. Effective clinical governance and risk management make it clear that quality is everybody's business.

Clinical governance, however, must not be seen as an end in itself; the aim is to move away from unacceptable variation in practice, but where there are justifiable differences in practice, to ensure that clinicians are accountable and responsible for these differences. This is a recognised part of clinical governance which does not aim to homogenise care.

Reference

See also KEY REFERENCES, piii

1. See also Walshe, K (1998) 'Cutting to the heart of quality', *Health Management*, vol 2, no 4, pp20–21.

Useful websites

National Institute of Clinical Excellence: *www.nice.org.uk*

Commission for Health Improvement: *www.chi.nhs.uk*

6 Managing health, safety and environmental risks

Dr Vanessa L Mayatt

This chapter covers:

- **The nature of health, safety and environmental risks in healthcare**

- **Risk assessment**

- **Legal requirements**

- **Corporate manslaughter and sentencing**

- **Learning lessons from incidents**

- **Best practice in managing health, safety and environmental risks**

- **Interface with clinical risk**

The first aim of this chapter is to enhance understanding of the nature and diversity of the health, safety and environmental risks associated with healthcare delivery. The second aim is to facilitate awareness of and the ability to use effective systems to manage these risks. In addressing these two main aims a range of associated topics will be covered, including hazard and risk, risk assessment, learning lessons from past incidents and the potential consequences of failure. The interface with clinical risk issues will also be explored, together with current legal and best practice requirements in relation to health, safety and environmental risks relevant to the healthcare sector.

Existing guidance

Existing guidance for the healthcare sector on health, safety and environmental risks is not in short supply. The Health and Safety

Commission (HSC) through its Health Services Advisory Committee (HSAC), and the Health and Safety Executive (HSE), have produced many documents which include general guidance on legal requirements and how to manage particular areas of risk relevant to the healthcare sector. The NHS and other organisations have also produced useful guidance. It can be confusing to successfully navigate a path through the plethora of existing guidance. The final aim of this chapter is to help to do so.

Health, safety and environmental risks in healthcare

The healthcare sector, in its broadest sense, includes hospitals (both NHS and private), ambulance services, diagnostic and research laboratories, post-mortem facilities, dental practices, GP practices, nursing and care homes, and office and teaching facilities. In a typical hospital, supporting the delivery of healthcare, are catering facilities, cleaning, building, plant and equipment maintenance, workshops, security, administrators and managers. Staff employed in the healthcare sector are therefore engaged in an extremely diverse range of work activities. Each of these work activities is associated with both common and differing health, safety and environmental risks. Some hazards present a risk not just for healthcare employees but also for patients, visitors and the environment. This can include radiation hazards, clinical waste and hazardous chemicals.

Commonly encountered risks

Individuals employed in the healthcare sector can be exposed to a broad range of risks that may result in harm. Eliminating or controlling these risks not only protects staff but is often the key to ensuring the safe and proper delivery of care. Commonly encountered risks are:

- manual handling
- hazardous chemicals and biological agents
- aggression and violence
- stress
- ionising and non-ionising radiation

Specific areas of risk

Particular work activities have their own attendant areas of risk. Examples include:

- **Waste disposal activities** – sharps, potentially infectious materials and manual handling risks

- **Theatres** – anaesthetic agents, X-rays, latex, ergonomic risks, manual handling, infectious agents and lasers

- **Post-mortem suites** – manual handling risks, hazardous chemicals, infectious agents, slips, trips and falls

- **Diagnostic laboratories** – hazardous chemicals, flammable materials, infectious agents, equipment and electrical risks

- **Wards** – aggression and violence, manual handling, stress, hazardous chemicals, infectious agents, drugs, slips, trips and falls

- **Facilities management** – construction activities, asbestos, electrical risks, hazardous chemicals, Legionella, transport, plant and equipment risks, flammable substances

- **Administrators and managers** – stress, aggression, violence, slips, trips and falls, display screen equipment and manual handling risks

- **Hotel service staff** – manual handling, slips, trips and falls, scalding risks, hazardous chemicals, machinery and equipment risks

None of the above examples contain an exhaustive list of all the ways in which risk may arise, as this depends on the precise circumstances in which work is undertaken and the nature of healthcare provided. Several groups of individuals may be exposed to risk which arises from a particular aspect of healthcare delivery, including staff, patients, visitors, seconded clinical and other staff, students (in teaching hospitals), and contractors.

How harm may arise

Food hygiene is an example of where there is the potential for large numbers of individuals to be exposed to harm. Food hygiene problems in hospital catering facilities have lead to outbreaks of food poisoning. Such incidents have the potential to affect staff, patients and visitors alike.

Table 1: Activity, risk and possible effect

Activity	Risk	Possible effect
HEALTH		
Anaesthesia	Inhalation of anaesthetic gases in theatres and recovery areas	Impaired behaviour and ability to work, depression of white cell formation, sensitisation of cardiac tissue, liver damage
Tissue preservation	Exposure to formaldehyde in pathology, histopathology and mortuaries	Chest tightness, coughing, occupational asthma, allergic dermatitis, sore throat, itchy eyes
Diagnostic imaging	Exposure to X-rays, ultrasound and electromagnetic fields	Cancer, hereditary defects, dermatitis
Invasive surgery	Exposure to body fluids and infectious agents	Hepatitis, tuberculosis, HIV, transmissible spongiform encephalopathy (TSE), latex allergy
SAFETY		
Nursing in care of the elderly wards	Exposure to physical and verbal abuse and manual handling	Stress, trauma, physical injury, musculoskeletal injury
Laundering of dirty linen	Exposure to cleaning agents, hazardous equipment and machinery	Skin sensitisation, physical injury, puncture wounds, scabies, hepatitis
Building and equipment maintenance	Exposure to hazardous equipment and machinery, working at heights	Physical injury, electrocution and falls
ENVIRONMENT		
High security isolation wards	Discharge to environment of infectious organisms	Exposure of members of the public and staff to infectious disease-causing organisms
Air conditioning and ventilation for healthcare premises	Release of bacteria including Legionella	Exposure of staff, patients, visitors and general public to organisms capable of causing life-threatening disease
Use of equipment containing mercury	Release of toxic chemicals from broken equipment	Exposure of staff, patients and the environment to a toxic substance during clean-up and disposal

A further example is a breakdown in infection control procedures – this can lead to widespread infection amongst patients and the staff associated with those patients. The consequences for patients who may be both susceptible to infection, for example, as a consequence of treatment with immunosuppressive drugs, and also very ill, can be very serious. Fatalities have resulted in the past from such incidents, and they are usually associated with a significant number of affected individuals becoming ill.

Looking in more detail at the nature of health, safety and environmental risks associated with healthcare delivery, reveals an almost bewildering array of ways in which harm may arise. Taking health, safety and the environment in turn, examples of how harm may arise are listed in Table 1.

Hazard and risk

Hazard and risk has been mentioned in a general risk management context in chapter 2. Within the health and safety arena, similar definitions for hazard and risk are also used. Hazard is an intrinsic attribute of a substance or situation. It is not therefore something that can be changed or altered.

Defining hazard and risk

HSE has defined hazard in guidance on risk assessment as "anything that can cause harm".[1] Hazard can also be described as the potential to cause harm. Harm includes injury, ill-health, damage to plant, equipment, property and the environment, and interruption to service delivery.[2]

Risk is the probability that harm will arise. HSE has defined risk as "the chance, high or low, that someone will be harmed by the hazard".[1] Risk therefore depends upon the precise circumstances to which individuals are exposed, their susceptibility and the extent to which risk is controlled. Risk is therefore something that can be changed.

Determining risk exposure

An example to illustrate this is nurses working in a children's gastro-intestinal surgery ward. Following major surgery, nursing such patients is associated with the hazard of manual handling. The extent to which nursing staff are exposed will depend upon:

- the weight and height of the children

- the extent of the patients' incapacity, or ability to move themselves

- the availability of patient moving and handling equipment, such as slides and hoists

- the training and encouragement of staff in the use of equipment and safe lifting techniques

- ward staffing levels

In this example, the risk of injury to staff will be higher with older (and hence heavier) children, grossly incapacitated patients and where no equipment or training has been provided. Irrespective of the patient, the provision of moving and handling equipment and training in its use will reduce the risk to staff.

The difference between hazard and risk

It is important not to confuse hazard and risk. Those who make the mistake of interchanging the two terms find that this can lead to confusion in risk assessment activities. It is quite possible to have a set of work circumstances where the hazard is high but the risk of harm arising is low. There are many examples to illustrate this point. Asbestos is a good example as it has the potential to cause death (from asbestosis, lung cancer and mesothelioma) and is therefore highly hazardous; however, the risk of harm arising will be low if:

- there is negligible asbestos in the working environment

- the asbestos-containing materials are in good condition or sealed in place so that no airborne particles arise

- the asbestos is inaccessible and is not scheduled to be disturbed

Risk assessment

Once the difference between hazard and risk is understood, the process of risk assessment is straightforward. Risk assessment is the basis of health and safety legislation, whether this concerns hazardous chemicals, manual handling, display screen equipment or more general requirements to manage risk.

Steps to risk assessment

Risk assessment is a structured process that is often described in a series of steps:

- hazard identification

- identification of who might be harmed and how

- risk evaluation

- documentation of risk assessment

- risk assessment review and revision

Example

Imagine a loading and unloading area at the rear of a central city hospital. The area is just off a main road with heavy vehicle use. Members of the public make extensive use of a footpath alongside the loading and unloading area. The area is used for the delivery of clean linen and other hospital supplies by different subcontractors. Deliveries are normally made by lorry.

In a corner of the loading area, containers are provided for the storage of clinical waste. Hospital staff deposit clinical waste bags in these containers daily. Clinical waste is removed for disposal by specialist subcontractors by lorry. Different subcontractors also deposit cylinders of medical gases, such as oxygen, helium and anaesthetic gases, into the area. A secure compound is provided for the gas cylinders but it is too small, so full and empty cylinders are propped up against the secure compound alongside which lorries drive in and out. Hospital staff use the loading and unloading area as a short cut to reach other parts of the hospital. Illicit parking by hospital staff and visitors in the area also takes place from time to time. Loading and unloading by subcontractors is mostly unsupervised by hospital staff.

Applying the risk assessment steps in relation to this scenario would reveal the information shown in Table 2 overleaf.

Measures to reduce risk

The whole point of risk assessment is making decisions about whether more needs to be done to remove or control risk. Risk assessments are therefore a means to an end and not an end in themselves. Many individuals, in carrying out risk assessments, fail to go the full distance and use the information gleaned during risk assessment to identify whether further improvement is necessary.

Going the full distance with the loading and unloading example, in other words identifying what needs to be done to remove or reduce risk

Table 2: Hazard, risk and nature of risk

Hazard identification	Risk to whom	Nature of risk
Moving vehicles	Subcontractors, staff, public	Physical injury, vehicle damage, property damage
Lifting and moving heavy objects	Subcontractors and staff	Musculoskeletal injuries
Falling cylinders	Staff, subcontractors, public	Physical injury
Damaged cylinders	Staff, subcontractors, public	Exposure to medical gases, physical injury, fire
Clinical waste	Staff, subcontractors, public	Fire, physical injury, infectious agents

(risk evaluation), would reveal a number of measures that could be taken to reduce risk. These measures would include:

- the provision of a one-way system for vehicles, speed limit signs and speed bumps

- marking out parking bays for lorries to use during loading and unloading

- demarcated footpaths

- signs prohibiting unauthorised access

- security supervision of the area

- provision of moving and lifting equipment

- relocation of a larger cylinder store away from moving vehicles

- prohibiting the storage of cylinders outside the cylinder store

- relocation of the clinical waste store so that hospital staff do not need to cross the loading and unloading area to deposit clinical waste

Legal requirements of risk assessment

In most instances it is a legal requirement to document risk assessments. It is also good practice to do so, otherwise risk assessments will not be incorporated into day-to-day activities and may need to be unnecessarily repeated. The function of documented risk assessments is not to be filed away and dusted off in preparation for a health and safety audit, but to be an integral part of routine work activities.

It is a further legal requirement for risk assessments to be reviewed so that they remain relevant and workable. Triggers for a review include accidents or cases of ill-health, organisational change, changes to working practices and new knowledge about risk.

Health and safety legislation requires risk assessments to be "suitable and sufficient". This necessitates that they address an assessment of all risks, consideration of the practicalities of preventing exposure and how risk can be removed or controlled.

Forms used in the healthcare sector for risk assessment are often overly long and complex, and require irrelevant information to be recorded. This usually leads to staff being reluctant to complete risk assessments, and therefore inadequate risk assessments. Health and safety legislation requires that risk assessments are carried out by competent individuals. Staff expected to carry out risk assessments need therefore to be trained and provided with supporting documented guidance and professional advice.

Stages of risk assessment

In order to successfully introduce risk assessment into an organisation or enhance the risk assessment process that is already in place, a sequence of stages needs to be worked through. These stages include:

Risk assessment policy

- Develop a short document setting out the organisation's aspirations on risk assessment and what is to be achieved. Good policies recognise the importance of prevention of risk, substitution with less hazardous alternatives and then risk control as a hierarchical approach.

- Responsibility for completion of risk assessments, review of risk assessments and taking action to effect improvements following risk assessment, should be clearly stipulated in the policy.

- The policy should be endorsed by the chief executive or organisational head and dated.

- Circumstances which would trigger a review of the policy should also be stipulated.

Development of a risk assessment form

- Aim for an easy-to-use form, ideally on one side of A4. If IT systems allow, a computer-based form can be used.

- Seek input from health and safety professionals, occupational health, risk managers, and other staff with relevant expertise on the layout and content of the form.

- Develop clear supporting guidance which staff can easily refer to when completing the form.

- Try out the use of the form and the guidance in different parts of the organisation, seek feedback from staff and amend the form and guidance as appropriate, prior to launching throughout the organisation.

- A key part of the form is indication of what action is required to be taken following risk assessment, by whom and when.

Risk assessment training

- Once responsibilities have been assigned within the policy, those nominated individuals expected to complete risk assessments will need to be trained to do so. This includes doctors, nurses and other staff.

- Training can be provided in-house if individuals are available who are themselves trained and qualified to do so. Otherwise external assistance can be sought.

- All those needing to be trained should be offered a training session.

- It is important to nominate representatives from all parts of the healthcare organisation for training, also for more complex risks.

- Effective training in risk assessment can be provided by a competent trainer in a few hours.

- Training sessions should be used to emphasise the importance of the organisation's policy, to provide specific training on the use of the risk assessment form and supporting guidance.

- It is vital that training includes practical case studies.

- It is good practice to follow up training sessions with further short workshops to enable staff to raise any practical problems encountered during risk assessment. The workshops need to be scheduled a couple of months after the original training.

- Refresher and retraining courses will be needed from time to time.

Many large healthcare organisations waste time and effort on risk assessment by not harnessing the expertise of their own staff. For example, laboratory and pharmacy staff typically have much experience of completing risk assessments in relation to hazardous substances. Their expertise can be usefully deployed in developing approaches to risk assessment throughout the rest of the organisation. Such staff often have access to risk assessment forms which can be used more widely. The overall aim should be to develop a single approach to risk assessment throughout the entire organisation. The use of both different assessment forms and different approaches to assessment in different parts of the organisation is to be avoided.

Legal requirements

Within the UK, health and safety legislation has been in place for around 200 years. This legislation has the aim of protecting individuals from harm arising from work activities. The early legislation was prescriptive and addressed specific areas of risk at work, such as dangerous machinery, lead and lifting equipment. In time this was followed by legislation that dealt with particular work processes, such as construction and chemical manufacture. The piecemeal nature of the legislation continued until fairly recently when legislation reflected a more holistic and logical approach to occupational risks.

The Health and Safety at Work etc Act

In 1974, ground breaking health and safety legislation was introduced, the *Health and Safety at Work etc Act*. This Act was different from all previous health and safety legal requirements as it was not specific to particular areas of risk, work processes or sectors of employment. It addressed for the first time the process by which health and safety should be tackled within organisations "to ensure the health, safety and welfare of employees". In particular, the Act had specific requirements for employers to:

- provide and maintain equipment and systems of work

- provide and maintain a safe working environment

- prepare a health and safety policy

- provide information, instruction, training and supervision

- provide adequate welfare facilities

Crown immunity

When the Act was first introduced, although it applied to hospitals and the healthcare sector, the Crown (including the NHS), was immune from prosecution. Crown immunity was, however, lifted in 1988 from the NHS so that the full bite of these legal requirements were felt by NHS hospitals and laboratories in the same way as they were by other sectors of employment. This late move of all of the healthcare sector under the umbrella of health and safety legal requirements, in comparison to other sectors of employment, was one of the reasons behind comparatively poor standards of health and safety in hospitals and other healthcare establishments at that time.

HSE powers

Health and safety legislation that applies to workplace activities, including the provision of healthcare, is criminal law. The legislation is enforced in healthcare premises (such as hospitals, care homes, GP surgeries, dental surgeries, health centres and clinics) by HSE inspectors. HSE inspectors have far-reaching powers which include:

- access to work premises at any reasonable time

- freedom to interview staff, contractors, visitors and patients

- taking of statements, photographs, measurements and samples

- confiscation of equipment and documents

- issue of notices (Improvement and Prohibition) requiring, respectively, improvements by a certain date or stopping a work activity until improvements are made

- initiation of criminal court proceedings for alleged breaches of health and safety legislation

Where cases are heard

Most cases involving contravention of health and safety legislation are heard in the magistrates' courts. Such cases are either heard by a stipendary magistrate or a bench of two or three lay magistrates. The maximum penalties that can be imposed by the magistrates vary according to the legislation involved; at the moment they range from £5,000–£20,000 or six months' imprisonment.

Crown court cases

Cases involving a more serious set of circumstances, such as a fatality or serious injury or a more serious breach of the legislation, may be referred to a Crown Court for hearing. The significance of this for defendants is that, if convicted, there is no limit to the penalty that a Crown Court can impose. In theory, therefore, higher fines may result in comparison to those set by the magistrates; in practice, however, this is not always the case. Cases involving breaches of health and safety legislation are known as triable either way – that is, both the prosecutor (HSE) and the defendant (the healthcare organisation or individual) can elect for trial in a Crown Court. In the past the prosecutor usually chose the venue, although some defendants selected a Crown Court as the venue, believing that a fairer verdict would be delivered by a jury.

In consequence of recent changes, defendants are now required to enter a plea (guilty or not guilty) and the courts then decide on the appropriate venue for the hearing. It is not unusual for Crown Court cases, particularly if they are defended, to last for several days or weeks. The associated legal costs can therefore be significant, but perhaps worth the risk to a defendant who truly believes they are innocent. It should, however, be borne in mind that HSE has an impressive track record in securing convictions for breaches of legislation. Defendants should therefore not make decisions lightly to defend the case or for the case to be heard in a Crown Court.

Defendants in HSE prosecutions

In most instances cases will be brought against the employing organisation, such as an NHS trust. A number of trusts have recently been successfully prosecuted by HSE for breaches of health and safety legislation. Prior to the creation of trusts, health authorities were also successfully prosecuted. The reason that most cases are brought against the employing organisation is that health and safety legislation confers extensive duties on employers. Investigation by HSE inspectors of either a workplace incident or during a routine visit or audit invariably identifies failures by the employer to meet legal requirements. A number of HSE prosecutions have, however, been taken against individuals, such as those engaged in running nursing and care homes.

Corporate manslaughter

At present there is active consideration of amending health and safety law to cover corporate manslaughter more properly. One of the drivers for this is the number of major incidents over the years involving multiple fatalities of members of the public or employees. Such incidents include:

- the 1987 Zeebrugge ferry disaster, 189 deaths

- the 1987 King's Cross fire, 31 deaths

- the 1988 Clapham Rail crash, 35 deaths and 500 injured

- the 1988 Piper Alpha fire and explosion, 167 deaths

- the 1999 Paddington rail crash, seven deaths and 151 injured

Investigation of these incidents has revealed a catalogue of corporate and individual failures.

The Paddington rail crash case

Following the Paddington rail crash, the train driver was indicted for seven manslaughter charges and a further case was brought against him for failing to discharge his duties as an employee under section 7 of the *Health and Safety at Work etc Act*. Great Western Trains were indicted for seven counts of corporate manslaughter and for failing to comply with section 3 of the Act. In the Paddington rail crash a high speed train en route from Swansea to London passed a red signal (a signal passed at danger or SPAD) which led to the train colliding with a freight train. At the time of the collision, the onboard safety system was inoperative.

In court, legal arguments centred around the negligence of individuals and determining the directing mind in an organisation. The judge hearing the case stated: "It is still necessary to look for such a directing mind and identify where gross negligence is that fixes the company with criminal responsibility."[3]

Calls for stronger legislation

This case, as have others before it, such as *R v P&O European Ferries (Dover) Ltd*[4] following the Zeebrugge ferry disaster, demonstrated the difficulty of securing corporate manslaughter convictions under existing legislation. This has led to calls for the existing legislation to be strengthened to enable more appropriate legal proceedings to be instituted.

A 1996 Law Commission report[5] recommended new legislation and a draft bill was prepared, to create new offences of reckless killing by gross carelessness and corporate killing, to replace the offence of manslaughter in cases where death is caused without the intention of causing death or serious injury.

Proposals for changing the law

In May 2001, the Home Secretary, Jack Straw, announced a consultation document on involuntary manslaughter and proposals for changing existing legislation. The proposals largely follow the earlier Law Commission recommendations but contain some significant differences. The proposals state that a corporation would be guilty of corporate killing if:

(a)   a management failure by the corporation is the cause or one of the causes of a person's death; and

(b)   that failure constitutes conduct falling far below what can reasonably be expected in the circumstances

If a corporate body is found guilty, it is proposed they will be liable to an unlimited fine. It is worth noting at this point the penalties that have been imposed in a number of recent cases where organisations and individuals were found guilty of breaches of health, safety and environment legislation.

Recent penalties for breaches

- In 1999, London Underground Ltd was fined £300,000 for breaches of section 3 of the *Health and Safety at Work etc Act* and the *Management of Health and Safety at Work Regulations*. The cases followed an accident where a passenger fell between the train and the platform at a Piccadilly line station.

- Following the Heathrow Airport tunnel collapse in 1999, Balfour Beatty was fined £1.2 million.

- The Environmental Agency secured a fine of £4 million against Millford Haven Port Authority following the leak of 72,000 tonnes of oil from the 'Sea Express'. The case was brought under the *Water Resources Act 1991*. Following appeal by the defendants, the fine was reduced to £75,000.

- In 2000, following an accident to an employee who was fatally injured when transferring waste into a tip, the owner of the company was sentenced to 12 months' imprisonment and suspended for two years.

If corporate manslaughter is introduced, it is a matter for debate and courtroom experience whether the legislation will have the desired impact – that is, to hold corporate bodies legally liable for serious accidents.

Breaches of professional duty of care where there is recklessness or gross negligence may also constitute manslaughter. A leading case[6] on this concerns an anaesthetist who during surgery failed to notice that the oxygen tube to the patient from a ventilator became disconnected. The patient suffered a cardiac arrest and subsequently died. The defendant anaesthetic was charged with involuntary manslaughter and convicted on the basis that he had been grossly negligent and there had been a gross derelection of care.

Death in relation to a work activity

Where death occurs in relation to a work activity, investigation into the circumstances is normally undertaken by the health and safety enforcing authority (HSE in the case of healthcare organisations) and the police. The focus of a police investigation is to establish whether the circumstances constitute manslaughter. The focus of an HSE investigation is to establish whether health and safety legislation has been complied with.

There have been several cases of manslaughter that have been tried in relation to patient fatalities. Cases of manslaughter have been instituted against healthcare employees, including consultants, where patients have died as a consequence of a medication error. These errors have arisen either due to alleged gross negligence on the part of the staff involved or due to intentional harm.

The increase in workplace fatalities over recent years is a further driver for corporate manslaughter. HSE figures for 2000/01 show a 34% increase in fatalities in comparison with the previous year. There are many, not just trade unions, who feel that the introduction of corporate manslaughter legislation is the most appropriate way to tackle this unacceptable tide of workplace deaths. It is, however, important to point out that under current plans it will not impact upon death caused by chronic exposure to, for example, hazardous chemicals or chronic injury from manual handling.

Sentencing

The leading case that is used for guiding sentencing of offences under health and safety legislation is *R v F Howe & Sons (Engineering) Ltd.*[7] This Court of Appeal case concerned a fatal accident to an employee of the company who was electrocuted whilst cleaning the appellant's factory with an electric vacuum cleaner. The cleaner was used to suck up water from the factory floor. The company had therefore failed to ensure the health and safety at work of one of its employees and "the lack of a system to check its electrical equipment fell far short of the appropriate standard."[8]

The judge hearing the appeal stated that penalties should be determined on a case by case basis. From that case, aggravating and mitigating factors which are now taken into consideration by the criminal courts in determining penalty include:

Aggravating factors:

- a failure to heed warnings

- whether a death has occurred

- whether a deliberate breach of health and safety legislation has taken place with a view to maximising profit

Mitigating factors:

- prompt admission of responsibility

- an early plea of guilty

- steps implemented to remedy deficiences and prevent a recurrence

- an otherwise good health and safety performance

It is expected that before trial, the prosecution and defence will agree on the aggravating and mitigating factors. This follows on from the case *R v Friskies Pet Care Co*[9] in 2000 where the court adopted the practice of the prosecution serving a list of aggravating factors and the defendant responding with a list of mitigating factors.

Whilst the maximum penalties that a court can impose are established, in practice the overriding criterion in establishing penalty is ability to pay. In consequence, courts often have difficulty in setting fines where the defendant is from the public sector, and are often swayed by the lack of financial reserves in NHS healthcare providers.

Main legislation

The main health and safety legislation in the UK remains the *Health and Safety at Work etc Act 1974*. This legislation forms the basis for all other occupational health and safety legislation.

Examples of health, safety and environmental legislation currently relating to the healthcare sector

Health and Safety at Work etc Act 1974

Management of Health and Safety at Work Regulations 1999

Control of Substances Hazardous to Health Regulations (COSHH) 1999

Manual Handling Operations Regulations 1992

Display Screen Equipment Regulations 1992

Personal Protective Equipment Regulations 1992

Ionising Radiation Regulations 1999

Electricity at Work Regulations 1989

Noise at Work Regulations 1989

Genetically Modified Organisms (Contained Use) Regulations 1992

Genetically Modified Organisms (Contained Use) (Amendment) Regulations 1996

First Aid at Work Regulations 1981

Consultation with Employees Regulations 1996

Safety Representatives Regulations 1977

Reporting of Injuries, Diseases and Dangerous Occurences Regulations (RIDDOR) 1995

Working Time Regulations 1998

Provision and Use of Work Equipment Regulations 1998

Lifting Operations and Lifting Equipment Regulations 1998

Workplace (Health, Safety and Welfare) Regulations 1992

Construction (Design and Management) Regulations 1994

Construction (Health Safety and Welfare) Regulations 1996

Control of Asbestos at Work Regulations 1987

Environmental Protection Act 1990

The *Health and Safety at Work etc Act* specifies the general duties of employers towards employees and others, which includes members of the public and patients in the context of healthcare delivery. It also specifies the duties of employees to themselves and each other.

Reasonable practicability

The duties are qualified by the clause "so far as is reasonably practicable". Reasonable practicability entails a balanced decision and that decision is based upon risk assessment. Reasonably practicable therefore depends upon:

- the degree of risk

- the time, trouble, cost and difficulty involved in removing or controlling risk

The amount of time, trouble and cost expended should not be grossly disproportionate to the risk. In demonstrating to HSE inspectors and proving to the criminal courts that reasonably practicable steps have been taken, clearly the greater the risk the more will be expected to be done to remove or control it. In meeting the test of reasonably practicable the principles of sound management and common sense need to be kept to the fore.

Management Regulations

In 1992, the implicit requirements of the *Health and Safety at Work etc Act* to manage risk were made somewhat more explicit by the introduction of the *Management of Health and Safety at Work Regulations*. These Regulations, usually referred to as the "Management Regulations" were updated in 1999. Like the 1974 Act, the Management Regulations apply to all work activities. A key part of the Regulations is a general requirement for risk assessment. Prior to these Regulations, the requirement for risk assessment was confined to legislation dealing with particular risks, such as hazardous substances, lead and asbestos. Further requirements under the Management Regulations relate to:

- making arrangements to implement health and safety measures

- appointment of competent advisers

- establishment of emergency procedures

- provision of information and training

- cooperation with other employers sharing the same workplace

The later requirement is particularly pertinent to healthcare organisations, where, for example, in large hospitals, employees of the trust or primary care group may work alongside university staff, out-sourced professional services, (such as occupational health) and Public Health Laboratory Service staff.

The consequences of failing to manage risks

The impact upon organisations and individuals of failing to manage health, safety and environmental risks can be very significant. The impact can include all or some of the following:

For organisations (employers)

- tarnished reputation
- loss of contracts
- delayed service delivery
- loss of key staff
- unplanned managerial time spent reacting to incidents
- court fines
- legal costs
- compensation claims
- high staff turnover
- increased insurance premiums

For individuals (employees)

- reduced capacity for work
- redeployment
- retraining
- reduced earning capacity
- early retirement
- death
- disability
- reduced quality of life
- loss of valued work colleagues
- imprisonment

The emotional impact

These lists, however, give little indication of the emotional impact of serious workplace failures to manage risk. No one expects their partner, family member, work colleague or friend to not come home at the end of the working day because they have been killed or seriously injured in a workplace incident. Whilst the percentage of the annual total of

---

Death by asphyxiation

In 1999, a research council employee working at a hospital died of asphyxiation. The individual had been filling containers with liquid nitrogen. He was already dead when he was found on the floor of the liquid nitrogen room by a colleague. This second employee fell in the room and struck her head whilst shutting off a liquid nitrogen bulk supply tank. She and her deceased colleague were subsequently dragged from the room by her supervisor. A total of five employees were admitted to hospital. It is not difficult to imagine that more than one member of staff could have died in this incident.

How the incident happened

The incident arose because of an unsafe system of work which was used during the liquid nitrogen filling process. A number of factors contributed to the depleted levels of oxygen in the filling room, including:

- inadequate extract ventilation to clear nitrogen from the room

- inadequate arrangements to allow for fresh air to enter the room

- inactivation of the oxygen alarm warning of low oxygen levels

- a leak in the liquid nitrogen storage tank allowing nitrogen to leak into the filling room

- lack of awareness amongst staff using the room as to the purpose of the oxygen alarm

HSE investigation

The HSE investigation of this incident concluded that several requirements of both the *Health and Safety at Work etc Act* and the *Management Regulations* had not been complied with. The employer was prosecuted by HSE and fined £25,000.

---

employee fatalities which occur in the healthcare sector is small in comparison with, for example, the construction sector, each fatality or serious injury is one too many. A recent fatal accident in a hospital illustrates the impact of workplace incidents (see box on previous page).

Learning lessons from incidents

Chapter 3 has addressed the importance of using incidents as learning opportunities. All incidents, whether involving actual harm or the potential for harm to arise, present opportunities to learn what went wrong and what needs to be done so that the incident does not arise again. This is as relevant in the management of health, safety and environmental risks as it is in other areas of risk management. Amongst health and safety professionals this is well-trodden ground as they have long used incidents in this way. It is worthwhile, therefore, looking at the specific impact on health, safety and environmental risks that incidents may present.

The Piper Alpha tragedy

In recent years one of the most major workplace incidents was the Piper Alpha tragedy in 1988. Following a major explosion and fire on the offshore platform, 167 workers lost their lives. A formal inquiry was held into the disaster in order to establish what had led to the incident. The inquiry uncovered a number of technical and organisational failures. In keeping with incidents in general, whether major or minor, a series of failures had occurred which led up to the disaster; rarely do incidents involve a single isolated failure.

The Piper Alpha inquiry identified error in maintenance procedures which eventually led to the leak which gave rise to the explosion and fire. The maintenance errors were attributed to inexperienced workers, poor maintenance procedures and poor organisational learning. There was a breakdown of communication on the platform and also to a sister platform which contributed to the scale of the incident. There was further breakdown in the permit-to-work system during shift changeover and safety procedures were insufficiently practised. The inquiry also revealed a number of human factor issues associated with the behaviour of individuals during emergency evacuation procedures and the ability of those in charge of the platform to retain authoritative control during a major disaster.

The accident pyramid

Piper Alpha was a complex disaster involving a series of failures which contributed to the precise nature of the incident and the devastating outcome. Major disasters such as this are, however, 'top-tier' events in an accident pyramid. Top-tier events do not occur every day whereas more minor incidents and near-misses can be commonplace. The important point is that the underlying root causes of minor incidents and major disasters can be the same. Chance plays its part in a series of failures coinciding and hence the final outcome. Risk management can do nothing to influence chance but it can identify and rule out failures and in so doing reduce the numbers of incidents which arise and the severity of their outcome.

Similar patterns of failure

Investigation of incidents arising within healthcare often reveal similar patterns of failure. Typically these include:

- a breakdown in communcation
- an absence of training
- lack of risk assessment
- lack of documented policy or guidance
- lack of resources
- conflicting demands placed on staff
- no monitoring of working practice
- lack of commitment to managing risk at the top of the organisation

The incident described earlier in which a research worker was asphyxiated illustrates a number of these failures. If there was a risk assessment for the nitrogen filling process, clearly it was not adequate. Staff were not trained in alarm and evacuation procedures. A further failure was in the provision of extraction and make-up air.

Learning opportunities

The learning opportunities from minor incidents or near-misses which do not result in harm should not be overlooked; they will be more numerous and if circumstances were different they could give rise to harm. Near-misses may also be more easy to investigate, as staff will be less concerned about their individual culpability.

Key lessons can be learnt about day-to-day working practices when incident information is combined with claims and complaints. A ward or department with a significant claims, complaints and incident history may be indicative of a fundamental management problem dependent upon the precise background, whereas an area of the organisation which has few complaints, a small number of minor unrepeated incidents and is associated with a high level of patient thank-you letters is likely to be in a different league in effective risk management.

Best practice in managing risks

Legislation contains minimal requirements for managing health, safety and environmental risks. Whilst compliance with legal requirements normally goes hand in hand with significant reduction in the numbers of workplace accidents,[10] any further improvement in performance entails going beyond legal requirements.

Many sectors of employment have developed their own specific responses to ensuring best practice in health, safety and environmental management. Such developments are often led by industry associations and other representative bodies, such as the Confederation of British Industry and the Chemical Industries Association. The healthcare sector is perhaps less fortunate than other sectors in that it does not have such long established representative bodies acting as the focus for the development of best practice. There is, however, nothing to stop risk management professionals in healthcare from looking at initiatives in other sectors to enhance performance and benchmarking in their own sector.

There is increasing evidence to indicate that these professionals are forming representative groups to take forward initiatives in the healthcare sector. Professional bodies IOSH and BOSH (Institution of Occupational Safety and Health and the British Occupational Hygiene Society respectively), both have specialist healthcare groups, facilitating networking amongst risk professionals and the sharing of experience.

Guidance available

There are numerous documented approaches available which can guide best practice in managing health, safety and environmental risks in healthcare. Unlike other sectors these approaches are less coordinated, so it is necessary to look in many directions to resolve the best way forward. Currently it is important to consider the following:

- controls assurance standards and supporting guidance

- guidance from HSC's Health Services Advisory Committee (HSAC)

- NHSE guidelines on health and safety issues

- HSE guidance *Successful Health and Safety Management*

- British Standard Institute guidance on health and safety management

- Guidance from the Department of Health, Medical Devices Agency (MDA), Advisory Committee on Dangerous Pathogens (ACDP) and Advisory Committee on Genetic Modication (ACGM) on health, safety and environmental issues associated with healthcare

- HSC Approved Codes of Practice on specific legal requirements

A route map through the guidance

A suggested route map through this plethora of best practice guidance is as follows:

- Legal requirements are not optional and as HSE, HSAC, ACDP, ACGM guidance is closely linked to legal duties and specific healthcare risks, start with these, and in particular the Approved Codes of Practice which have been developed in association with specific legislation and set out the route to compliance.

- HSE's *Successful Health and Safety Management* is a crucial document to use in the development of approaches to best practice, so move onto this next.

- Then move on to the closely related HSAC guidance on *Management of Health and Safety in the Health Services,* as this translates the previous HSE guidance for the healthcare sector.

- If general help is still needed on developing best practice approaches, consider the British Standard, but in real terms this adds little to the HSE and HSAC guidance.

- Once a general approach has been developed, supplement this with approaches to managing specific areas of risk by using HSE, DoH, MDA, ACDP and ACGM guidance as appropriate.

New developments

Keeping up to speed on new developments in best practice is a task that needs to be undertaken on a routine basis. One of the easiest ways to do this is by searching the websites of relevant organisations. A number of commercial organsiations also produce CD-ROM and software-based information which is regularly updated with new legal and best practice requirements. Some of these incorporate particularly useful word searches to help identify key guidance from all the main organisations. It is, however, important to understand the relative hierarchy of all the best practice guidance in order to develop a meaningful approach that does not involve wasted effort.

Keeping up with government thinking

In 1999, deputy prime minister John Prescott announced an initiative with a number of aims in the health and safety arena. He proposed:

- a strategic appraisal of the health and safety framework

- a new agenda for the first 25 years of the new millennium

- reducing the impact of health and safety failures by 30% over 10 years

This was followed in June 2000 by the launch of *Revitalising Health and Safety*.[11] The background to this document was a deeply held concern for the number of deaths in the workplace and the associated societal costs, which were estimated to be £18 billion per year.

Targets

One part of best practice in managing health, safety and environmental risks is therefore currently to comply with the targets set in the *Revitalising* document. Unlike other sectors, these targets are not generally uppermost in the minds of healthcare managers and risk management specialists. They are nevertheless key targets to work towards. Targets for Great Britain have been set by the Government to:

- reduce working days lost per 100,000 workers from work-related injury and ill-health by 30% by 2010

- reduce incidence rate of fatal and major injuries by 10% by 2010
- reduce incidence rate of work-related ill-health by 20% by 2010
- achieve half the above by 2004

These targets lend further importance to the need to have effective incident recording systems and analytical arrangements in place. Without such systems it is impossible to set targets and know when they have been achieved. In organisations where there is no maturity in incident recording systems, as is the case for many healthcare providers, the introduction of targets for accident reduction can be counter-productive and merely drive down reporting levels. Thorough planning and careful communication within the organisation is therefore necessary if this particular aspect of best practice is to succeed.

Further motivations for achievement of best practice are currently being considered by the Government. These include:

- linking court penalties for breaches of health and safety legislation to turnover or profit
- prohibition of directors' bonuses for a fixed period
- suspension of managers without pay
- suspended sentences pending remedial action

In July 2000, HSE produced *Securing Health Together*[12] which set out its occupational health strategy for England, Scotland and Wales. The strategy adds detail on occupational health targets following the earlier *Revitalising* document. Specific targets for achievement by 2010 are:

- a 20% reduction on the incidence of work-related ill-health
- a 20% reduction in ill-health to members of the public caused by a work activity
- a 30% reduction in the number of working days lost due to work-related ill-health

Whilst targets, particularly in the long neglected area of occupational health, are important, many organisations will find these distinctly 'un-SMART'. Most organisations, including those in the healthcare sector, have no accurate data on occupational ill-health and the second target is particularly challenging for the sector, where patients die whether despite best efforts or because of a failure in care. Cynicism apart, these HSE targets should be viewed as a spur to improving the health at work of employees and ensuring that arrangements are in place to prevent exposure to risks to health.

Using available expertise

One key part of securing best practice concerns the use that is made within organisations of available expertise. Most large organisations, including those in the healthcare sector, have access to in-house risk management expertise. Rarely is it the case, however, that the in-house health and safety and occupational health provision expertise is deployed to maximum effect. In order for best practice to be achieved such expertise needs to be given the credibility that it deserves. All too often, however, these risk professionals are to be found way down in the organisation's hierarchy.

Proactive use of in-house expertise is also important in pushing towards best practice standards. Risk management expertise, including health, safety and environmental specialists, should not just be consulted when there is a problem, but when plans and developments are being considered so that problems can be avoided.

Establishing effective systems

Prior to the publication of HSE's *Successful Health and Safety Management* in 1991,[2] a specialist part of the HSE had spent over 15 years carrying out detailed reviews of health and safety management systems in an extensive number of employing organisations. Many of these organisations were at the leading edge in terms of effective systems to manage health, safety and environmental risks. The 1991 HSE guidance therefore reflected in some detail what organisations in practice did to achieve enviable health and safety performance. This background is important to appreciate because it adds to the weight of this particular HSE publication. The guidance describes a five-step management system (Figure 1).

The steps in the system constitute an iterative process which is repeated over time in order to secure progressively better performance. The steps are similar to general approaches developed more recently in relation to controls assurance and corporate governance. Health and safety professionals have been known to debate where in the loop an organisation needs to start. It is, however, fair to say that in the absence of policy, an organisational structure and plans, it is not possible to carry out the successive parts of the loop in a meaningful

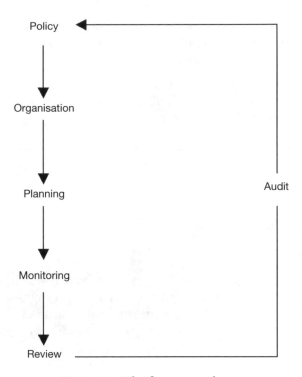

Figure 1: The five-step cycle

way. It therefore makes sense to start with policy and work through the other steps in a logical fashion.

A typical situation

Anyone who has stepped into a risk management role within a healthcare organisation will, however, know from experience that typically:

- Some policies exist, but they are not up to date, the chief executive has forgotten to sign them, and many parts of the organisation have never seen them. Others have seen them but do not follow them.

- Some semblance of an organisational structure is in place, but there is often lack of clarity about the roles of groups and individuals, so that much effort is duplicated and other issues are not addressed at all.

- Health and safety planning consists of reacting to events that happen, and earmarking a percentage of the budget for health and safety but failing to prioritise how the money is spent.

- Monitoring performance is normally reactive and only consists of reviewing recorded incidents. Active monitoring of achievement of planned objectives is rare.

- Performance review is rarely done in-house and most usually involves consultants, CNST assessors, NAO staff, financial auditors or HSE inspectors.

With some effort, this scenario can be turned around so that the healthcare organisation drives its health and safety programme rather than the other way round!

The five-step process

Policies

These do not need to be lengthy documents which cover every conceivable angle. Many multinational organisations employing thousands of people throughout the world succeed in producing health, safety and environmental policies which cover no more than one side of A4.

Aim for a short general policy document which sets out the organisation's overall aspirations and key responsibilities of individuals.

The general policy can be supplemented by other policies dealing with specific areas of risk such as infection control, laboratory work, and directorate policies. Some points to remember are:

- The policy should be signed by the organisation head, dated and regularly reviewed.

- It should recognise that health, safety and the environment is central to high quality service delivery, reducing costs and looking after staff.

- Be wary of including large slices of legal requirements in a policy document as this is meaningless in conveying aspirations.

- Include positive statements about why health and safety is important.

- Make sure that the policy can be read and easily understood by all groups of staff.

Forward-looking health and safety policies reflect the need to develop people and become an integral part of ensuring organisational success and effective staff development. Policies increasingly recognise the continuum between work life and non-work life and that an individual's performance, and in consequence that of the employing organisation, is affected by work and non-work experiences.

Organisation

The overall aim should be to implement the health and safety policy and to facilitate the move to better performance.

Good organisation involves assigning responsibilities to those members of staff with key health and safety responsibilities and also groups, such as the health and safety committee, risk management group and manual handling coordinators.

Organisational arrangements need to ensure that:

- The organisation drives its health and safety programme – not the other way round.

- Cooperation is encouraged and not hampered.

- Staff are competent and undertake roles assigned to them.

- There is effective communication from the top down, the bottom up and throughout all layers of the organisation.

Planning

This should be viewed as the means by which priorities and objectives are established in relation to health, safety and environmental risks. Risk assessment and incident analysis are a key part of planning, in order that priorities are properly set. Planning is about proactivity and deciding what to do next on the basis of available evidence.

Effective planning requires resources to be assigned, teamworking and a desire to see progress happen. It requires determination and commitment. Objectives for improvement need to be SMART: specific, measurable, achievable, realistic and time-bound. A good test of effective planning is to ask whether there is an overall plan for health, safety and environmental issues and whether the right priorities are indicated in the plan.

Monitoring

Monitoring progress and measuring performance are key steps in ensuring increasing improvement in performance over time. Health and safety professionals often categorise monitoring systems as either active or reactive. Incident recording is in essence reactive monitoring; active monitoring is more concerned with the achievement of plans. Examples of active monitoring of progress include:

- attendance by staff at a risk assessment training course

- appointment of manual handling coordinators

- refurbishment of the gas-scavenging system in theatres

In other words, active monitoring is about checking achievement of specific objectives in the health and safety plan.

Review and audit

The previous four steps form the main plank of a health and safety management system, but it is important to check that the system is having the desired effect in terms of health and safety performance. This brings us to the review step. This step encompasses the use of audits, of which there are many in the health and safety arena.

Many organisations outside of the healthcare sector place regular reliance on health and safety audits to verify their performance. These audits are either carried out in-house or by external consultants. Some audits are paper-based, others software-based. Some have been developed specifically for the healthcare sector. In purchasing a proprietary audit package, of which there are several, it is important to establish that the audit is relevant and is capable of being repeatedly used over a period of time. This is a specialist area and one where the views of health and safety colleagues should be sought.

Interface with clinical risk

When the healthcare sector first started to give priority to risk management, clinical and non-clinical risk tended to be separated. There were a number of reasons for this. Different individuals, particularly within hospitals, were responsible for these areas. The absence of a coordinated risk management strategy also contributed to the separation. Clinical risk tended to be regarded as the preserve of clinicians, and non-clinical risk the responsibility of others.

Within hospitals the use of different incident recording systems to record clinical and non-clinical incidents, and the fact that the number and nature of these incidents were rarely combined for scrutiny, also played its part. The healthcare sector lost valuable ground in dealing with risk management by allowing clinical and non-clinical risk to be separated. Within the health and safety profession in general there is considerable expertise in incident recording, analysis, trend spotting, root cause analysis and implementing change when things have gone wrong. This expertise can be deployed in looking at incidents in general, including clinical incidents. Even now in many parts of the healthcare sector the separation between clinical and non-clinical risk still exists. The DoH's report *An Organisation with a Memory* (see KEY REFERENCES, piii) and the diversity of expertise tapped into during the preparation of the report clearly illustrate the benefits of involving risk experts from outside the clinical arena.

Recent HSE prosecutions

Over the last couple of years, there have been a number of prosecutions taken by HSE inspectors as a consequence of hospital incidents. On first examination these incidents would appear to be clinical incidents in which patients have either been harmed or even killed. The HSE has, however, succeeded in demonstrating to the criminal courts that health and safety legislation nonetheless applies, and healthcare providers have been accordingly convicted of breaches of this legislation. This has further called into question the wisdom of separating clinical and non-clinical risk.

One case that illustrates the lack of wisdom in separating clinical and non-clinical risk is an HSE prosecution which followed the death of a patient undergoing a cardiac angiogram. The patient died because air was injected into their body, rather than contrast medium. None of the staff involved in the procedure checked that contrast medium was in the equipment prior to starting the pump. HSE considered that this was a breach of section 3 of the *Health and Safety at Work etc Act* as the trust had failed to secure the health and safety of others (a patient). The court agreed with HSE, and the trust was found guilty and fined.

The important point about this case is that many lessons can be learnt not just in relation to clinical practice, but in relation to managing risk more broadly. The successful HSE prosecution serves to underline the importance of looking at incidents and risk management in general on a more holistic basis.

References

See also KEY REFERENCES, piii

1. HSE (1998) *Five Steps to Risk Assessment*, Health & Safety Executive, London.

2. HSE (1997) *Successful Health & Safety Management*, Health & Safety Executive, London.

3. *R v Great Western Trains* [1999] unreported

4. *R v P&O European Ferries (Dover) Ltd* [1991] 93 Cr. App. R72

5. Law Commission (1996) *Involuntary manslaughter: Law Commission report 237*, Law Commission, London.

6. *R v Adomako* [1994] 4 All ER 935

7. *R v F Howe & Sons (Engineering) Ltd* [1999] 2 All ER 249

8. Forlin G (2001) *Corporate killing: where are we now?* Proceedings of the 2001 IOSH Conference.

9. *R v Friskies Pet Care Co* [2000] 2 Cr. App. R(S) 401.

10. Mayatt VL (1996) 'The management of occupational health and safety', *Health Care Risk Report*, vol 2, no 10.

11. HSE (2000) *Revitalising Health and Safety*, Health & Safety Executive, London.

12. HSE (2000) *Securing health together*, Health & Safety Executive, London.

Further information

Health at Work in the NHS (*www.hawnhs.hda-online.org.uk*)

BMA (1994) *Environmental and Occupational Risks of Healthcare*, BMA publishing, London.

HSE (1998) *Guide to Risk Assessment Requirements*, Health & Safety Executive, London.

HSE (1996) *The Costs of Accidents at Work*, Health & Safety Executive, London.

HSE (2001) *Occupational Exposure Limits*, Health & Safety Executive, London.

Health Services Advisory Committee (1997), *The Management of Occupational Health Services for Healthcare Staff*, HSAC, Luton.

7 Managing the physical environment

Trevor Payne

This chapter covers:

- **The healthcare physical environment**

- **Estates and facilities management**

- **Contracting for facilities management service delivery**

- **Facilities operational risk: pressure systems, maintenance, fire, and electricity**

- **Security of staff and assets**

- **Training and development**

The physical or built environment is increasingly being recognised as a vital component of the provision of effective healthcare. There are more than 700 safety-related statutes in the UK, and approximately 100 of these are of day-to-day concern to those providing services and running facilities management and estates functions in healthcare establishments.

In addition there are over 100 authoritative codes of practice – and with guidance constantly growing or being updated, it is vital that facilities staff are kept well briefed on statutory compliance and risk management. There are a large number of statutory issues affecting facilities management (FM), along with a number of controls assurance standards (see KEY REFERENCES, piii). This chapter will outline some of the major areas for property-related statutory compliance, and key aspects of facilities risk that relate to FM services and the physical environment.

The provision of healthcare is a holistic process which combines the three elements of people (staff), process (work patterns, routines, systems) and workplace. Clearly the physical environment (building or hospital) needs to support the activity or process that takes place within it and be fit for purpose, whilst providing an environment that is warm, comfortable, clean, attractive and safe for staff, patients and visitors. A therapeutic and supportive physical environment can have a positive effect on recuperation and also the morale of patients, staff and visitors.

A varied environment

The physical environment in which healthcare is delivered can vary greatly in terms of size, age, design, decorative order and condition. Modern hospitals and healthcare establishments are designed and built in line with Health Building Notes which provide guidance on the design and layout of specialist areas and infrastructure to support effective service delivery, such as intensive care units and theatres. Clinical links and departmental interdependencies are now considered at the design stage in new healthcare developments, in order to ensure that typical patient journeys are taken into account.

The patient journey

The patient journey details the route map that the patient follows during a particular episode of treatment, and outlines all of the areas, services and clinical specialties that they encounter until the episode is completed. This approach takes into account typical patient flow patterns, maps contact with specialist departments and establishes how often, where and when the patient encounters these services.

By taking into account these regular and routine interactions the hospital can be designed or redesigned in such a way as to support typical patient journeys. This in turn avoids unnecessary patient movement, and logistical problems where staff and vital equipment have to be moved around the hospital or find themselves inappropriately located. Older healthcare premises may have been developed without full consideration to the patient journey or interdependency.

The challenge of older buildings

Due to the changing nature of healthcare delivery methods, a large number of hospitals and healthcare premises have outlived their original design concepts, and are not suitable to support the provision of modern healthcare services which are high-tech and highly serviced. This presents risk relating to service provision.

The NHS has the largest property portfolio in Europe comprising some 1,200 hospital sites worth around £23 billion. Sixty-five per cent of the estate is over 35 years old, with a large number of Victorian and listed properties. A large amount of the NHS estate was not designed to support today's methods of healthcare delivery. The NHS Plan (see KEY REFERENCES, piii) sets a target that 40% of the total NHS building stock will be less than 15 years old by 2010, and 25% of the NHS maintenance backlog will be cleared by 2004.

A large amount of the NHS estate has significant backlog maintenance and robust risk management is required in order to manage risk relating to issues such as fire safety, Legionella, asbestos, or electricity. There are also a number of other risk factors that need to be addressed – business risk, service continuity, outsourcing, procurement of services and contract management all fall into this important category.

Old or new, the property, people and process combination needs to be carefully and effectively managed with respect to risk, and health and safety. Risk needs to be assessed and managed in the buildings in use, the processes or work methods followed, and the management of staff, patients and visitors within the healthcare environment.

Estates and facilities management

The term 'facilities management' is a relatively new concept to healthcare. There is no standard model of service provision, so the basket of services managed under the FM umbrella and the links to the trust board vary widely. The growth of FM in UK healthcare over the past decade has been rapid and far-reaching. The facilities profession has developed from its early formative stage in the late 1980s, through a rapid growth phase during the 1990s. It is reaching a level of maturity and credibility which will guide it through the first decade of the new millennium.

Facilities service contractors

Similarly, the majority of facilities service contractors have gone through a metamorphic change over the last few years. Many companies have been acquired by or merged with large construction firms, while large-scale professional cleaning contractors have acquired catering contract companies with the aim of extending the basket of services that they can offer. The overall result has been the emergence of a 'super league' of facilities providers who can cover the broad remit of healthcare facilities and estates management.

These service providers are able to service a wide market apart from healthcare, including sectors such as education, defence and local government. Some of these FM providers are now poised to take on global FM. They are also positioning themselves as consortium partners for the Private Finance Initiative and Public/Private Partnerships – deals that will secure contracts for periods of 25–40 years.

The professionals involved

The evolution of FM has involved professionals from a varied collection of professional disciplines in the management of facilities services. Property and the built environment play a key role and this has required the professional skills of architects and quantity surveyors. The way that people interact with the built environment has required the input of human resources professionals and the technical expertise of building services and maintenance staff.

The processes that take place within buildings such as catering, cleaning, security, or the mailroom have required practical operational management from a range of specialist professional backgrounds – not to forget the overriding management of risk across all of the disciplines. This varied assortment of professional and management skills, coupled with pressure to downsize the organisation and to flatten management hierarchy, has spawned a new breed – the facilities manager.

The new breed of facilities manager

The new breed of facilities manager is likely to be responsible for a range of services outside their original professional discipline. It is commonplace for those who used to be quantity surveyors, architects, maintenance engineers, office managers, catering managers and human resource managers to now be responsible for the delivery of the full range of facilities services in their organisation. Facilities managers have by necessity become generalists not specialists. This, however, should not in itself present a risk management or service management issue. Healthcare FM is after all predominately a management function – which achieves its results by harnessing the effective output from people, property and process.

Defining FM

Many definitions of FM exist but they are all variations on a theme. The following definition of FM, from NHS Estates, will be used and expanded upon in this chapter:

> "The practice of coordinating the physical workplace with the people and work of an organisation; [FM] integrates the principles of business administration, architecture, and the behavioural and engineering sciences."

A core function

The traditional view of FM has been that of a non-core or pure support function which is often seen to be at arm's length to the main thrust or activities of the organisation. From a risk management perspective, it is vital that each organisation understands the importance of facilities services and fully considers the services it deems to be core and non-core to its operation.

Certainly, in the early days of FM, much emphasis was placed upon facilities taking control of and managing all of the non-critical or non-core functions – which would then enable the organisation to focus on the main business agenda and the core issues that it might be facing. Clearly there are benefits associated with combining the management of support functions under one umbrella. Additional benefit is achieved by breaking down traditional demarcation boundaries and combining service functions in an innovative manner – cutting out duplication and wasteful practice.

The extent of FM

Many organisations are now beginning to realise the true potential of FM services and recognise that they are more than just pure support functions limited to operational service delivery. The evolving nature of FM and the maturity of its approach has begun to ensure that a strategic FM dimension is now a requirement for all successful and forward-thinking organisations.

If all the functions of a healthcare organisation were to be analysed and the processes involved portrayed as a supply chain, then a number of key links in the chain would be provided and managed by the facilities function. In its best operational mode, FM could be described as the glue that holds the organisation together. The FM span covers tasks achieved by basic manual handling at one end of the spectrum, through to hi-tech, highly-serviced electronic medical devices at the other.

Facilities strategy

As FM has evolved and developed within organisations, there has been a steady realisation of the benefits (tangible and intangible) that can be obtained from effective management of FM services. If facilities professionals are to be truly regarded as players within the organisation, then it is essential for the facilities manager to develop a facilities strategy. This should map over a stated period of time how FM services will be reviewed, re-engineered or moulded to best support the needs of the organisation.

The strategy should ideally comprise three strategic elements that build upon the current level of provision and should map short, medium and long-term goals and targets and give direction for facilities over the stated period. If the strategy is to be of any real value then it must reflect the aims and ambitions of the organisation that it is designed to support. The facilities strategy must clearly complement the overriding business strategy, and this can only happen if the senior facilities professional is in tune with the vision of the organisation.

A thorough approach to risk management underpins service delivery and should be outlined in a way that is clearly understood in the facilities strategy. As the organisation evolves over time the strategic direction may need to be modified to take account of external influencing factors, which will require emergent strategy to be developed – this approach may also mean that elements of strategy remain unrealised (Figure 1 opposite).

The developed strategy must, however, take account of the core business of the organisation and its own corporate strategy, direction, mission and values. If FM is to develop in harmony with the organisation that it supports, then it must develop a degree of strategic alignment and focus upon shared values. Also, more importantly, the facilities manager must become a part of the

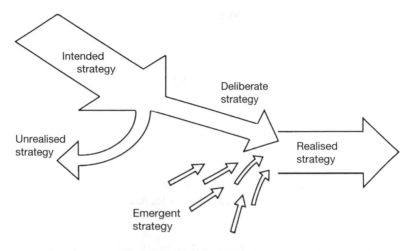

Figure 1: Strategy development

decision-making body (that is, a board-level player) if facilities are truly to become proactive and to ensure that the full risk impact of facilities-related issues are considered.

Facilities risk

Facilities risk can be focused into two specific areas:

- **Strategic risk** – risks associated with procuring service contracts, including outsourcing and in-sourcing decisions.

- **Operational risks** – risks associated with day-to-day operational provision of a range of facilities services, many of which are covered by statutory legislation and guidance.

Contracting for facilities management

European procurement process

Public procurement law states that any public service contract with a sum total in excess of the relevant threshold must comply with European Union General Agreement on Tariffs and Trade (GATT) legislation when going out to the market to test services. Compliance with the EU Directive on public procurement is mandatory. Its Directive is to promote and maintain competition in public procurement within the EU, to control restrictive practices, and to try to create a level playing field for potential contractors competing for work.

There are three procedure options:

- restricted
- open
- negotiated

Restricted procedure

Restricted procedure is most frequently used within the NHS, and enables the selection of tenders to be controlled. The contracting authority invites interested parties to show Expressions of Interest and from the received expressions a selected group is invited to tender.

All contracts exceeding a stated threshold value (currently over £100,000 excluding VAT) must be advertised in the *Official Journal of the European Community* (OJEC) for a period of 37 days prior to the Invitation to Tender. Tenders must be issued for a period of not less than 40 days to those responding within 48 days of a contract award, and notification must be placed in the OJEC. Selection of tenders from those responding to the advertisement must not discriminate on grounds of nationality. Criteria for exclusion are specific and organisations must be able to demonstrate fairness in the selection process.

Open procedure

Open procedure is also available but is less frequently used, as it allows all of those expressing an interest to receive tenders and has a longer period (52 days) for receipt of Expressions of Interest.

Negotiated procedure

Negotiated procedure involves direct discussion and negotiation between supplier and procurer in order to arrive at a final offer. This procedure requires careful consideration as it attracts ministerial attention, and there needs to be clear reasons why the negotiated route has been chosen over the open and restricted options. It is therefore only available in limited circumstances.

Exemptions to the procedures

Bearing in mind the purpose of the legislation, exemptions are limited and strictly defined. In the case of genuine urgency (failure to plan ahead is specifically excluded) an accelerated procedure may be allowed – an example might be the sudden and unforeseeable failure of a critical piece of equipment, but not an unexpected release of funds.

Where appropriate, the period for receipt of Expressions of Interest may be reduced to 15 days and the tender period to 10 days.

Non-compliance

Where suppliers feel that they have been unfairly disadvantaged they are encouraged to seek redress through the Compliance Directive (a section of the EU Directive on public procurement). Therefore in any circumstances where a supplier is excluded from competition, the reasons must be set down and must be applied equally to all suppliers.

The Government requires an annual return from all public bodies showing the value of business placed within and outside the Directives. Failure to comply with the legislation is likely to be noticed.

The decision to outsource

The decision to outsource elements of an organisation's facilities activity or support service delivery is a major strategic decision. The ultimate decision must be based on confidence that the service provider can deliver a consistent, affordable, high-quality service in accordance with the specification, whilst demonstrating synergy with the future strategic direction of the host organisation. The decision will be based upon a key set of circumstances usually focused around cost, quality, service delivery and risk – unique in each instance and for each organisation, often with each factor weighted to reflect impact and importance.

Clearing dead wood

Charles Handy wrote:[1]

> "Organisations are responding to the challenge of efficiency by exporting unproductive work and people as fast as they can."

It is true to say that some of the early outsourcing decisions were made for all of the wrong reasons. Rather than tackling or managing issues relating to lack of flexibility, generic working methods or rigid demarcation boundaries, many organisations outsourced what they considered to be inflexible and uncooperative departments and service functions.

In so doing, unruly management and supervision were transferred to the outsourced provider for them to manage and control. For many organisations, outsourcing was initially seen as an opportunity to clear the dead wood and reduce headcount, fuelled by a trend towards downsizing. The decision to outsource may also have been influenced by a focus on the complexity of day-to-day service issues without perhaps considering some of the longer-term issues.

Careful consideration

What do organisations gain from outsourcing? The decision to outsource or in-source must be thoroughly considered and evaluated before a decision is made. Outsourcing or in-sourcing can have a demoralising impact on staff groups and result in a reduction of output and productivity in the short term.

If the original decision to outsource was wrong then this may lead an organisation to consider bringing the service back in-house. Often by the time this point has been reached, a considerable pool of labour, expertise, loyalty and knowledge has been lost as a result of the initial transition and this will make returning to in-sourcing more difficult. This does not make it impossible, but there will undoubtedly be a time lag whilst the service re-establishes itself and expertise is developed. A hump of costs associated with setting up human resources, payroll, management and supervisory structures will be incurred as systems are put back into place.

Core versus non-core

The core versus non-core discussion should be considered in the outsourcing debate, in order to determine the services that the organisation retains or manages in-house. Careful consideration needs to be given to identifying those services that are best managed directly by the organisation.

A strategic view must be established on the importance of each service element when it comes to risk and business continuity. It is important to identify knowledge in each service area, to establish the value of that knowledge and to gauge how difficult it would be to replicate each function. It is therefore vital that the functional linkages and service boundaries that exist between departments and directorates are identified and mapped, before any contract bundle or service package is assembled prior to outsourcing.

Talk over lunch

In most organisations there are often casual arrangements in place between departments to resolve minor issues, such as discussion of minor problems over lunch. This interaction happens on an informal but regular basis and is never in the specification for the service, and as a result it becomes a variation to contract. Some companies have found out too late that they have mistakenly outsourced core services.

Meeting the customers

In the facilities context there are potential problems with outsourcing services that bring the contractor face to face with the customers of the service. Kotler and Bloom define service as:[2]

> "any activity of benefit that one party can offer to another that is essentially intangible and does not result in ownership of anything. Its production may or may not be tied to a physical product."

Services are performances not objects, and staff therefore need to be trained to give the correct performance for a variety of audiences. Contract staff need to be proficient in customer care and able to handle difficult situations as they arise.

Service specification

A lot of the early attempts at outsourcing failed due to poor specification. Often specifications were ill-prepared and incomplete, resulting in post-contract variations and escalating costs, or alternatively specifications were so detailed and complicated that it scared contractors off. There has been a shift away from detailed input specifications that are said to limit or stifle innovation towards output specifications that are less prescriptive and focus on the required service output.

Contract relationship

Often organisations have found out too late that they have exported valuable knowledge and expertise, which is difficult to place a price on and even more difficult to replace once it has been lost. That expertise and knowledge represents power and now it sits with the contract provider.

This shift of power is often exploited in the contract scenario in order to add leverage to decisions relating to extending the contract. The contractor will assess the competence of the informed client or the contracts manager during the mobilisation stage of the contract. If they know more about the outsourced service than the client, and if the knowledge and expertise has been transferred to the contractor as a result of outsourcing, then the contractor is placed in a very powerful position. This power shift may in itself be a spur to in-source the service and develop expertise, particularly if it is considered to be in an area of core activity. A decision to in-source based on this scenario will often be difficult, time-consuming and have high switching costs – but it is not impossible to achieve.

Supplier leverage

Supplier leverage can be demonstrated in a number of ways such as:

- price hikes
- withholding access to new technology
- a reduction in the quality of work produced

Lonsdale and Cox summarise the factors which lead to supplier leverage as follows:[3]

- **Poor contracting** – issues that are known within the firm are omitted from the contract. Either inappropriate personnel are assigned to the task of closing the deal, or the personnel concerned have inappropriate priorities.

- **Limited supply market options** – the firm chooses to outsource despite there being a limited number of supply options available to it.

- **High asset specificity** – because of the highly specific nature of the investment a firm makes in an outsourcing relationship, there is an effective absence of competition at the end of the contract period.

- **Uncertainty** – in situations where a firm has made highly specific investments, it will be even more vulnerable to supplier leverage if the nature of transaction between the buyer and the supplier is characterised by uncertainty. Uncertainty will lead to an incomplete contract, which will in time give the supplier the opportunity to charge excess fees.

When things go wrong

If outsourcing has failed to deliver, for whatever reason, it is important to revisit and dissect the circumstances and reasoning behind the original decision to outsource, and establish exactly why the process did not work, before making a kneejerk decision to in-source or revisit the market. Establish the current position before launching into a potential solution. It is essential that the way forward dovetails with both the facilities and the host organisation's strategy.

Analysis

Factors to consider when analysing the original decision are:

- In-house versus outsourced supply – re-visit the original decision to outsource.

- Core or non-core activity – does the service represent core activity?

- Service specification and contract – was the specification robust, relevant and kept up to date with requirements? Was there a contract in place?

- What benefits were perceived and what benefits were received?

- Contract management and performance monitoring – how effectively was the service monitored against the specification?

- Organisational change – people, process, and workplace.

- Contract relationship – power and leverage.

Service delivery

There are no off-the-peg solutions to the provision of FM. The portfolio of services and the range of options relating to the various combinations of service delivery have sparked discussion and debate over their respective merits.

Options include:

- in-house versus contract service provision, as discussed earlier in the chapter

- Single-service or single-source contracts versus multi-service contract clusters, or total FM (TFM) contracts where one contractor manages and controls the entire facilities portfolio

The risk here centres on economy of scale and knowledge within the organisation. Is it best to procure and manage a number of small and potentially quite demanding single-service contracts for a range of services, or to go for the one-stop shop approach? Each organisation needs to consider whether it has the time and expertise to manage single contracts and what the benefits of TFM might be to them.

The ultimate decision on the approach to take will depend on the organisation's unique requirements. One size does not fit all.

Changing fashions

Each approach will have risk attached to it, and advantages and disadvantages that need to be fully considered. The late 1980s and early 1990s were the era of the changing organisation, where 'out' was in, organisational hierarchy and management structures were flat and the customer was king. The traditional model of the organisation as it previously existed has been remodelled – its hierarchy and structure have been pulled apart, re-shaped and re-assembled, thus ensuring each component part is necessary and required and adds value to the delivered product or service.

Seamless service delivery

There has been a steady move away from the traditional methods of service delivery that in the past served to protect and support the practice of operating within controlled trade demarcation boundaries. These boundaries or service interface points between trade groups, staff groups, and contractors are steadily being eroded as service providers strive for the seamless approach to service delivery. It is in this remodelling that one of the key benefits of the facilities approach lies. Stripping out the inflexible barriers of demarcation can allow true innovation in how services are provided, and with this approach inefficiency can be eliminated.

Individuals can have more rewarding and more satisfying jobs that provide interest, flexibility and a degree of staff empowerment. True success in this approach rests in effective training, and clarity in the definition of role boundaries. The risks associated with multi-skilling and generic working need to be fully considered and comprehensive training, support and orientation provided to ensure that services are delivered in a safe and appropriate manner.

Obviously some factors, such as a change in statutory compliance requirements, will force strategic priority to be reconsidered. Once a strategy has been developed and objectives set it does not mean that a blinkered view must be taken.

Facilities operational risk

A number of the statutory issues relating to FM services concern services and service infrastructure, which are often described as behind-the-scenes services.

These issues include:

- facilities risk management
- pressure regulations
- good practice in equipment maintenance
- risk assessment for homeworkers
- fire safety
- electricity at work
- security of staff and assets
- training and development

These topics will be dealt with in turn below.

Facilities risk management

Health and safety legislation

Both employers and employees have a legal responsibility with respect to health and safety. It is essential that facilities managers, either in-house or outsourced, understand health and safety legislation and their duty of care, and put systems in place to comply with the legislation. It is vital that all facilities contractors are aware of the risks associated with their contracted place of work and of their own legal duties.

It is also essential that the facilities manager is satisfied that contractors comply with health and safety legislation and supporting guidance, and have conducted risk assessments. Routine monitoring of health and safety systems and procedures is recommended, and a compliance clause with respect to health and safety must be drafted into any specification or service level agreement (SLA). Good health and safety awareness and practice is a critical success factor for any organisation.

Health and safety legislation confers specific duties on employers, those in control of premises and employees to ensure health and safety at work. There are specific requirements for risk assessment. Risk assessments have to be robust, comprehensive, appropriate and kept up to date. Where there are five or more employees, significant findings of this assessment have to be recorded, and employers must draw up a health and safety policy statement and bring it to employees' attention. The requirement for a policy and risk assessment is fully explored in chapter 6.

Risk assessment systems

There is an element of risk in all activities. Risk assessment is designed to identify high-risk activities and to ensure that safe systems of work are designed and adopted in order to minimise the risk. Each year about 1.1 million employees suffer workplace injury. This injury rate results in the loss of an estimated 30 million working days at a cost of £900 million a year to industry. Add to this extra costs to social security and the health service, and the loss of income by the victims, and the estimated overall total cost comes between £10–£15 billion per year.[4] Properly conducted risk assessment should reduce the likelihood of workplace injury and ill-health.

There are a number of paper-based and software systems designed to assist in the risk assessment process. Key areas to consider when conducting a workplace risk assessment relating to a task or activity include:

- air quality and temperature, water systems, pressure systems

- electricity, fire, noise, asbestos and hazardous substances

- lighting, trailing leads, glass openings, doors and gates, and mobile work equipment

- staff facilities, personal protective equipment, visual display units and manual handling

- first aid, sanitation and washing facilities
- disability access

Pressure Regulations

The main Regulations covering pressure systems and pressure equipment are the *Pressure Equipment Regulations 1999* and the *Pressure System Safety Regulations 2000*. The failure of operational pressure equipment or pressure systems – resulting in the uncontrolled release of pressurised agents – could kill or seriously injure people nearby and cause considerable damage to property.

Typical pressure systems

In a healthcare setting, examples of typical pressure systems and equipment are as follows:

- pipework and associated hoses
- autoclaves and pressure cookers
- steam systems, including steam traps or filters, and valves
- boilers
- compressed air systems
- pressure gauges and indicators

The main reasons for pressure system failures are:

- poor installation, design and equipment specification
- poor maintenance and system repair
- unsafe work systems
- operator error, poor supervision and training

Failure of a pressure system can cause the following:

- fire – due to the uncontrolled release of chemical, whether liquid or gas
- impact from flying debris or equipment parts, or blast impact
- contact with released contents of the pressure system – steam or gas

Avoiding pressure system failure

A series of measures can be put into place in order to reduce the risk of pressure system or equipment failure. These are:

- Design the system and install it in accordance with appropriate standards, specifications, guidance and Regulations.

- Ensure that safety devices are installed.

- Regularly inspect the system/equipment and maintain it at the required frequency – using suitable materials and spares.

- Develop and adopt a safe system of work.

- Provide appropriate training on the system for all relevant staff.

- Develop operating procedures and clear working instructions and ensure that they are kept updated. The operating instructions should include the operating condition of the product under pressure (for example, gas) and instructions for dealing with emergency conditions.

- If the system is extended or altered ensure that the training, maintenance procedures, spares and operating instructions and plans are updated to reflect the changes and the requirements and condition of the changed system.

Examination of pressure systems

A written scheme of examination drawn up by a competent person is required for all pressure systems, except those classified as exempt in Schedule 1 of the *Pressure Systems Safety Regulations 2000*. Pressure systems must not be used without having a written scheme of examination. The written scheme must cover all pipework, vessels and protective devices.

Good practice in equipment maintenance

In many organisations the maintenance equipment and the physical environment forms the backbone to the facilities remit – perhaps because many facilities managers have a building or engineering background. Maintenance will undoubtedly form a major part of any SLA or contract when it is included in the facilities remit, but FM is not about being an expert in all areas or professional disciplines.

Therefore, maintenance does not necessarily have to be managed or controlled by an estates professional. In many organisations the facilities team may be very lean and expert advice is bought in as and when required. This can also apply to estates consultancy, as in some organisations, the entire range of estate-related services has been outsourced to the contract sector.

It is perfectly feasible for a personnel, human resources or facilities manager with a catering background to have responsibility for site maintenance within their total facilities remit. There is a mystique surrounding the management of maintenance that it is riddled with risk and statutory obligation to such an extent that it 'must' be managed by estate professionals.

Statutory obligation and risk management do indeed form key components in the safe and effective management of estate and property; however, the key is to ensure sound back-up and advice on maintenance, either from within the FM team or from an independent consultant on a retainer.

Outsourcing maintenance

It is preferable to keep the advisory role separate from the maintenance contract, as a sharp operator will identify areas of weakness and vulnerability and could exploit them. However, it may be equally desirable to outsource the provision and management of maintenance to a contractor completely – in which case the facilities manager needs to identify the budget and the specification and leave the delivery and innovation to them. In this scenario, agreement on the specification and monitoring systems is vital.

The specification must be comprehensive and include plant asset lists, life cycle costing definitions, schedules of rates for repair works, cost threshold levels, and so on. The final decision will be unique to each organisation. The method of service delivery will greatly depend on the size of the organisation, the scale of the FM function and economy of scale with respect to contract bundling of services.

Types of maintenance

This section will briefly outline the management of planned and unplanned maintenance with a view to minimising risk relating to maintenance and operations.

The definitions of various types of maintenance, taken from British Standards, are as follows:

- **Maintenance** – the combination of all technical and associated administrative actions intended to retain an item in, or restore it to, a state in which it can perform its required function (*BS 3811: 1984*).

- **Maintenance programme** – a time-based plan allocating specific maintenance tasks to specific periods (*BS 3811: 1984*).

- **Breakdown maintenance** – the operation of restoring an item to a state in which it can fulfil its original function after a failure in its performance (*BS 8210: 1986*).

- **Corrective maintenance** – the maintenance carried out after a failure has occurred and intended to restore an item to a state in which it can perform its required function (*BS 3811: 1984*).

- **Emergency maintenance** – the maintenance which it is necessary to put in hand immediately to avoid serious consequences (*BS 3811: 1984*).

- **Repair** – restoration of an item to an acceptable condition by the renewal, replacement or mending of worn, damaged or decayed parts (*BS 8210: 1986*).

- **Remedial work** – redesign and work necessary to restore the integrity of a construction to a standard that will allow the performance of its original function (*BS 8210: 1986*).

- **Planned maintenance** – maintenance organised and carried out with forethought, control and the use of records, to a predetermined plan based on the results of previous condition surveys.

- **Condition-based maintenance** – preventative maintenance initiated as a result of knowledge of an item's condition gained from routine or continuous monitoring (*BS 3811: 1984*).

- **Preventative maintenance** – maintenance carried out at predetermined intervals, or corresponding to prescribed criteria, and intended to reduce the probability of failure or performance degradation of an item (*BS 3811: 1984*).

The above list could be divided into two groups – planned (programmed) maintenance and unplanned (response) maintenance. This brief outline is intended to define these two types of maintenance and to highlight the need to offset the peaks and troughs of unplanned maintenance with planned work. In this way responsiveness to the unknown and unplanned can be balanced with statutory compliance, service requirements and frequencies.

Planned and unplanned maintenance

Unplanned maintenance can be broken down into a further two categories:

- normal response
- emergency response

Planned maintenance can similarly be broken down into:

- preventative
- cyclical

Service delivery

Critical systems (such as nurse call, power supplies, or a renal water treatment plant) and their associated service response and rectification times will need to be outlined in the SLA for each location. The helpdesk (see below) can be utilised to generate data that relates to requests for maintenance and repair of these systems, and this data enables a comparison between actual (time from request to repair) and stated SLA response and rectification. This approach will highlight performance, and areas where resources should be targeted in order to maximise the availability of labour, spares and consumables.

Maintenance systems operated as part of a helpdesk or computer-aided facilities management (CAFM) system usually work on a job ticket or docket system. Dockets or requests are issued to contractors or tradespeople. These will include details of the location, a description of the fault and an agreed response time. Some also include an allowance for or estimate of the time required to complete the repair. Planned maintenance dockets may have the service routine printed on the docket to aid the tradesman. The request or docket will also include a cost code used to log all labour costs and spares or consumables used during repair or maintenance. Goods will generally only be issued against a request or docket and they are immediately coded against the cost code for recharging purposes.

Effective logging

Some contracts or SLAs operate against a schedule of agreed rates (costs per hour) for breakdown maintenance with spares used in repairs charged extra to contract. In theory all consumables used during a planned service should have been quantified and included in the contract or SLA. Some of the more sophisticated maintenance software systems have bar codes printed onto the dockets, to enable the completed job requests and supplies requisitions to be scanned straight into the computer in order to log labour hours and materials, thereby cutting down on the amount of manual data entry required. It is vital that all planned requests or job dockets are completed and fed back into the system in order to collect costs, response times, materials used and status of repair.

The system can also be used to log plant history and maintenance frequency – this is important for statutory maintenance tests for pressure vessels or electrical installations. By following this type of approach to maintenance, it will ensure that as far as possible systems and equipment are maintained in accordance with manufacturers' recommendations and that all maintenance tasks are recorded along with spares used and the details of the person carrying out the task. This provides a full service history. It is also important to log when planned routines have been rescheduled or pulled forward – perhaps to take advantage of downtime or a shutdown – to ensure that the number of planned maintenance visits stated in the specification or the SLA are delivered.

Planned preventative maintenance

Planned preventative maintenance (PPM) is usually programmed on a cyclical basis. For example, a heating system will need to be maintained under PPM at the following frequencies:

- weekly
- six-weekly
- quarterly
- half-yearly
- yearly

A maintenance routine will be drawn up that takes into account the manufacturer's service requirements, replacement frequency and any local implications. A series of tasks or checks will be scheduled against the PPM frequencies. Six-weekly tasks include the weekly tasks plus some additional checks or service requirements; quarterly tasks include the six-weekly tasks, and so on.

Planning ahead

In order to plan workload and manpower resources, all of the PPM maintenance frequencies need to be entered into the maintenance program or work planner. The program will look at all of the site's PPM tasks over a year and highlight where there is a clash of routines – perhaps 20 quarterly routines have been programmed for the same week, which it would not be possible to resource.

Most maintenance programs have a feature that allows workload to be planned over a given period to achieve best fit with available resources plus an allowed percentage for unplanned response. For example, a maintenance department could base its operations on a ratio of 70% PPM to 30% unplanned or repair work. If this were the case, an estimate of the total PPM hours required for the stated workload over the year could be used to establish the level of manpower or resources required to service the specification or SLA, with a buffer of generic working to ensure 100% utilisation of the labour pool in a productive manner. While there is some flexibility to offset peaks and troughs of demand and planned/unplanned workload, some maintenance tasks are statutory (equipment must be inspected and results documented at stated frequencies) and therefore must be completed at the defined PPM frequencies. In addition, maintenance of large boiler plant, pressure vessels and lifts will have an insurance implication and will need to be inspected during maintenance by an appropriate insurance engineer.

Effective maintenance

The following steps are essential in order to effectively manage maintenance:

- Identify and comply with any statutory obligations.

- Identify and assess all risks.

- Produce a detailed asset register of all plant and equipment.

- Produce a comprehensive specification (input or output).

- Develop safe systems of work based on risk assessments of all tasks.

- Identify key components or items of equipment vital to business continuity and prioritise maintenance tasks/spares.

- Develop a PPM schedule for key items of plant and equipment.

- Provide appropriate training and support for maintenance staff.

- Record and document maintenance performance and test results.

- Agree a process and a specification for a helpdesk or work requisitioning/scheduling system.

- Agree a schedule of rates for unplanned maintenance.

- Communicate with other parts of the organisation.

Note that capital investment appraisal and life cycle costing are not included in the above list. It is assumed that the elements of life cycle costing – including purchase, installation, commissioning, operation, spares, consumables and disposal – have all been fully considered prior to asset purchase as part of the investment appraisal. Therefore planned maintenance costs and training or familiarisation have been budgeted for before the asset is put to use and requires maintenance support.

Risk assessment for homeworkers

With the ready availability of reliable and relatively inexpensive data and telecommunication technology, more and more staff are choosing to work from home if their work patterns and duties allow it. The *Workplace (Health, Safety and Welfare) Regulations 1992* do not cover the home although an employer's duty of care to protect the health and safety of their employees still applies regardless of where they work.

Most responsible employers will either carry out a home-based workplace risk assessment or will have an assessment audit tool that home-based employees can complete themselves. The assessment should cover a range of standard items such as:

- lighting

- electrical power and socket requirements

- fire safety

- storage space, the working environment and ergonomics

- security

- display screen equipment

- fire safety

Fire precautions and risk assessment

The legal requirements with regard to safety from fire where people are employed to work are, in the main, one or both of two pieces of legislation:

- The *Fire Precautions Act 1971*

- The *Fire Precautions (Workplace) Regulations 1997*

Guidance

Specific guidance on fire engineering in hospitals and healthcare establishments is available from the suite of 17 documents that make up *Firecode*.[5] Each of the documents focuses on specific applications relating to fire. Three of the main documents are:

- *Health Technical Memorandum (HTM) 81 – Fire precautions in new hospitals*

- *HTM 85 – Fire precautions in existing hospitals*

- *HTM 86 – Fire risk assessment in hospitals*

The *Building Regulations 1991 (Approved Document B)* detail the fire safety measures required in new buildings and buildings which are to be extended or structurally altered.

A specific safety standard is also included in controls assurance (see KEY REFERENCES, piii), which sets out a number of fire safety criteria by which to measure fire safety performance. The criteria mirror both mandatory and statutory obligations along with best practice guidance.

Health Service Circular

Health Service Circular 1999/191[6] set out the ministerial priorities with respect to fire engineering in healthcare establishments. The circular states that:

- No patient area is to be in an unsafe condition – that is, no areas to remain in estate code condition D – by 31 March 2001, or an outline business case to support improvement is to be in place to support this initiative.

- Backlog work is to be eradicated by 31 March 2003.

This circular has served as a focus for fire safety improvement and provides a non-negotiable end point for eradication of the fire safety backlog by early 2003.

Fire engineering and design

HTM 81 provides guidance relating to fire engineering and design in new hospital buildings and takes into account important fire issues such as escape, evacuation, and compartmentation – that is, control of the spread of fire. It is vital that fire engineering is considered at the design stage. The local fire service and the planning authority will take particular interest in applications relating to the design and upgrade of healthcare establishments.

HTM 85 provides guidance on similar issues to *HTM 81*, but is focused on upgrade, retrofit and overcoming inadequacy in the fire engineering elements of design components of existing buildings.

Annual fire risk assessment

An annual fire risk assessment must be carried out in all areas of a hospital.

The assessment should cover the following areas, as required by *HTM 86*:

- **Hazards** – ignition sources such as smoking, arson, equipment, and work processes. This will identify if the trust has a no-smoking policy, localised risks of arson, and location and storage of potentially hazardous equipment such as gas bottles. It will also highlight potentially hazardous work practices carried out in the locality, such as welding.

- **Combustible materials and surface finishes** – this covers the presence of significant potential fire load and expanses of varnished wood panelling, furniture, and fabrics.

- **Precautions** – fire prevention measures, fire barriers, and smoke dampers.

- **Communications** – alarm and detection systems, and zone plans.

- **Means of escape** – fire exits, escape routes and signage.

- **Containment** – structural elements, fire compartmentation and fire protection to hazard areas.

- **Extinguishment** – availability and suitability of fire-fighting equipment.

All of the above are scored as being either:

1. high standard

2. acceptable risk/hazard or *HTM 85* standard

3. high risk/hazard

4. very high risk/hazard

5. inadequate

6. unacceptable

Balancing life risks, hazards and precautions

HTM 86 provides an approach to risk assessment based on balancing life risks, fire hazards and existing fire precautions. Regular fire risk assessment needs to be carried out and should not just focus on active and passive fire detection, but also identify local issues that may cause fire problems, such as clutter in fire escape routes, the risk of arson, storage of combustible materials or medical gas cylinders.

Some healthcare buildings may require fire certificates. This requirement will be dependent, for example, on the design and layout of the building, the number of staff in the building and the work process taking place in the building. Discussion should take place with the local fire authority to determine which buildings they consider should have fire certificates. Staff should be made aware of the fire-related risks pertinent to the area that they work in. This awareness should cover passive and active fire detection, fire-fighting equipment location and its appropriate use, and fire signage/escape route and evacuation procedures.

Electricity at work

Statistics indicate that there are about 1,000 accidents at work involving electric shock or burns each year that get reported to the HSE. Around 30 of these are fatal. Most of these fatalities arise from contact with overhead or underground power cables. There are basic but effective measures that can be adopted in order to control the risks relating to the use of electricity at work.

Main hazards

The main hazards are:

- contact with live parts causing burns and electric shock (mains voltage can kill)

- explosion or fire where electricity could be the potential source of ignition in explosive or flammable atmospheres

- electrical faults that could cause fires

In order to reduce the risks associated with electricity, the risks must be identified by a full risk assessment. This identifies the hazards, evaluates the risk arising from the hazards and identifies who might be harmed as a result and how. The risks associated with the use of electricity at work are amplified when electricity is used in surroundings, which are:

- **outdoors** – perhaps outside of the electrical zone of protection

- **wet** – which under certain circumstances could cause unsuitable equipment to become live

- **confined or cramped** – particularly when working in tanks, bins or silos involving close proximity to large surface areas of earthed metalwork which make it difficult to avoid shock

Reducing risks

Risk associated with electricity can be reduced by:

- **Reducing the voltage** – such as portable power tools running at 110 volts, temporary lighting operating at a reduced voltage or in some circumstances the use of battery powered tools or air/hand powered tools.

- **Maintenance and inspection** – it is essential to ensure that existing electrical installations are safe and are regularly maintained so as to keep them in a safe condition.

- **Conforming to standards** – new electrical installations should be designed in accordance with the Institution of Electrical Engineers wiring regulations and installed to a suitable standard such as *BS 7671 – Requirements for electrical installations and associated guidance notes*. This standard does not have statutory power but provides a useful indication of good industrial practice in meeting the *Electricity at Work Regulations 1989*.

- **Testing** – electrical installation and testing is now being linked to a new specific section of the Building Regulations and this move will see a structured and formalised approach to regular testing of installations – carried out by specialist testing professionals. Installations should be regularly maintained and tested for safe operation. Testing should also include a visual inspection to identify damaged or fraying power leads, or overloaded power sockets. Fixed installations should be tested periodically by a competent person; records of these periodic tests are useful for plant history and for assessing the effectiveness of the installation.

- **Provision of safety devices** – it is vital that electrical circuits have adequate and effective protection afforded by circuit breakers, fuses, or residual circuit breakers. As electrical distribution systems are extended or adapted to meet current demand requirements, the type and rating of the circuit protection must be checked in order to ensure that the type of protection provided is still appropriate. It is also important to ensure that circuit overload and rating of the protection is correct, in order to protect the installation and the users, and that circuit discrimination is maintained. The protection device closest to the fault should operate first.

- **Suitable equipment** – equipment must be suitable for the environment in which it will be used and must be maintained regularly in order to ensure that it is safe and functioning correctly. It is good practice to keep a list of all electrical equipment, portable tools and appliances and record test results.

- **Safe working systems** – ensure that people who are working with electricity are competent to do so. Work on or near exposed live parts must not be allowed unless it is absolutely unavoidable and suitable precautions have been taken to prevent injury, both to the workers and to anyone else who may be in the area. Thorough risk assessment must be undertaken and documented outlining why it has been assessed as unavoidable to work on or near to exposed live parts.

Security of staff and assets

Security of staff and assets is everyone's responsibility, but there is very little in the way of legislative requirement to provide security. The only statutory requirements to take security measures are either:

- general duties to provide a safe and healthy place of work for employees

- specific requirements where there are issues of national patient security or where explosives or dangerous substances are being stored

There may also be contractual responsibilities requiring employers to protect people and assets. Where equipment is required to maintain the safety of employees, such as a closed-circuit television (CCTV) system for staff working in a potentially vulnerable location, this is covered under the *Provision and Use of Work Equipment Regulations 1998*. It should be noted that the *Data Protection Act* also contains specific requirements relating to the management of CCTV systems. Employers may wish to impose a confidentiality agreement as part of the employment contract in healthcare establishments.

Security needs to be considered as part of a wider approach to risk management, which addresses risks to people, property and the business. Most healthcare establishments have systems in place to cover bomb threats, suspect packages, business continuity, and fraud (as discussed in chapter 8) and this demonstrates that security-related risks have been assessed in part. However, security management in healthcare establishments is a growing area of risk that needs to have focus and high visibility.

Zero tolerance

The NHS has taken a hard-line, zero tolerance approach to crime and violence in hospitals, where staff can be subjected to physical or verbal abuse from patients, their families and the public. This is no longer generally tolerated and must not be accepted as part of the day-to-day consequence of providing healthcare. However it is not just those working in accident and emergency or staff at the acute end that are subject to abuse – often reception staff and staff working in areas with public interaction, such as outpatients, restaurants and portering, that face security problems.

Risk assessment, training in defusing aggression or conflict resolution, physical barriers or secure design approaches and CCTV can minimise these risks. Many trusts have implemented sophisticated ID badge and access control systems to assist in security management in healthcare establishments; these systems can be used to manage staff, visitors and contractors. There is always a trade-off in hospitals between ease of access and the need for security, and this trade-off will impact in different ways at each site.

A local solution must be sought following a thorough risk assessment that looks at the building and the way it is used. Risk assessment should also identify lone working practices. An important aspect of the assessment is to to identify areas that may become a target for theft, such as cash handling offices, or areas where computers or attractive consumables are stored. A security strategy complete with operating policies and procedures relating to the risks identified will assist in the management of these risks, and will aid communication with staff.

Training and development

Training and development is an area that has been overlooked in the past with regard to facilities staff. All too often staff are unable to be released from their dpay-to-day operational duties, or cannot be covered by colleagues during training sessions. It is in the interests of both employer and employee to ensure that appropriate and timely training is given and received. Indeed given the frequency of new and updated statutory legislation and guidance, it is vital that staff are kept abreast of new requirements, guidance and techniques.

Recruitment and retention

A major risk facing many healthcare employers (particularly those in the South of England where unemployment is low and healthcare salaries are uncompetitive) is recruitment and ongoing retention. Employers need to be creative with the employment package on offer if to attract and keep the right staff. Training should not therefore be limited to statutory updates or an annual fire lecture. Employment packages do not solely consist of pay – the opportunity for training and development may also be attractive to staff. The importance of professional development is dealt with in chapter 9. The skills and competencies of each member of staff should be assessed, to inform a structured training and personal development plan. This should contain updates on health, safety and statutory issues.

What should training include?

Training can be provided initially during staff induction and orientation and basic fire safety training – looking at the location of fire exits, fire fighting equipment, and break glass points. General organisational policies such as infection control, clinical waste segregation, and security should also be provided. It is also beneficial to demonstrate to staff the sound of fire and other alarms. Basic lifting and handling training should be provided tailored to the activity that the employee carries out. Information regarding the control of substances hazardous to health and workplace risk assessments should also be explained to new starters so that they are made fully aware of risk in their workplace and of the procedures in place to identify and minimise those risks. Health and safety training requirements are more specifically discussed in chapter 6.

Giving staff further responsibilities

Over time as staff become familiar and comfortable with the workplace they could be encouraged to take on responsibility for specific areas of risk management in their locality, such as becoming the local fire marshal, local health and safety representative, or the local back care trainer. Appropriate training will need to be provided to support these duties but this approach leads to broader awareness of specific and general aspects of risk management in the workplace, and encourages a sense of ownership for workplace health and safety.

At given periods, staff with specific technical training – such as the medical gas authorised person, high voltage/low voltage electricity authorised person, steriliser engineers, or catering staff – will need to have a refresher or update course. It is important that employers therefore treat staff training and development seriously and manage the process of delivery.

A methodical approach

This chapter has outlined the importance, scale and complexity of risk relating to the physical environment and the operational aspects of supporting healthcare delivery. It has been shown that due to the diverse nature of service delivery and premises, a proactive but methodical approach is required in order to identify and deal appropriately with risk in this dynamic environment.

Management of these risks needs to link into the strategic view of the organisation in order to identify and consider the impact of actions implemented to manage or reduce an area of risk. Facilities managers also need to be in a position to provide advice and guidance on the risks associated with changes to service delivery. Risk also needs to be effectively managed across the virtual organisation that makes up the facilities team – comprised of contractors, project workers, architects and outsourced service providers. The trust's authorised officer needs to be certain that contract partners have a robust grasp of risk management, consistent with the trust's overall approach to managing risk.

References

See also KEY REFERENCES, piii

1. Handy, C (1994) *The Empty Raincoat*, Hutchinson, London.

2. Kotler, P and Bloom, PM (1999) *Marketing Professional Services*, Free Press, New York, USA.

3. Lonsdale, C and Cox, A (1998) *Outsourcing: a business guide to risk management tools and techniques,* Boston, Earlsgate.

4. Unpublished research conducted by Trevor Payne.

5. *Firecode*, NHS Estates (tel: 0113 254 7299 or *www.nhsestates.gov.uk/property_ management/content/fire_code.html*).

6. Health Service Circular 1999/191 (*www.doh.gov.uk*).

Legislation

Pressure Equipment Regulations 1999

Pressure Systems Safety Regulations 2000

Provision and Use of Work Equipment Regulations 1998

Safety of Pressure Systems: Pressure Systems and Transportable Gas Containers Regulations 2000. Approved Code of Practice

Building Regulations 1991 (Approved Document B)

Control of Asbestos at Work Regulations 1987

Fire Precautions (Workplace) Regulations 1997

Fire Precautions Act 1971

Workplace (Health, Safety and Welfare) Regulations 1992. Approved Code of Practice and Guidance

HSE Guidance

Check the HSE website for the most up-to-date guidance at *www.hse.gov.uk* or call the HSE infoline on 08701 545500. HSE Information Services, Caerphilly Business Park, Caerphilly CF83 3GG.

HSE (1998) *Five steps to risk assessment*

HSE (1998) *Electrical safety and you*

HSE (1993) *Electricity at work – safe working practices*

HSE (1994) *Essentials of health and safety at work*

HSE (1994) HSG 107: *Maintaining portable and transportable electrical equipment*

HSE (1994) *Written Schemes of Examination*

British Standards

(1984) *BS 3811: Glossary of Maintenance Management Terms*, British Standards Institution, London (*www.bsi-global.com*).

(1986) *BS 8210: Guide to Building Maintenance Management.*

(1992) *BS 7671: Requirements for electrical installations and IEE wiring regulations: guidance notes.*

Further reading

Barrct, P (ed.) (1996) *Facilities Management: Towards Best Practice*, Blackwell Science, Oxford.

British Institute of Facilities Management (1999) *Survey of facilities managers' responsibilities*, BIFM, Saffron Walden. (*www.bifm.org.uk*)

NHS Estates (1996) *Re-engineering the Facilities Management Service*, Health Facilities Note 16.

Payne, T (2000) *Facilities Management – a strategy for success*, Chandos Publishing, Oxford.

8 Service continuity management

Graham E Offord

This chapter covers:

- **The definition of service continuity management**
- **The nature of disasters in healthcare**
- **The impact of service interruption**
- **Developing service continuity plans**
- **Implementation of service continuity plans**
- **Resourcing service continuity management**
- **Strategic benefits**

Within risk management circles, the concept of business continuity management is not new and is applied with varying degrees of rigour in commerce and industry.

In the service sector, however, the use of the term 'business continuity' does not sit comfortably with many professionals. The services they provide are not for profit, and are normally delivered in accordance with best practice and value for money. Accordingly, the term 'service continuity' tends to be used.

Either term encapsulates the philosophy of establishing a way of working that will ensure service delivery regardless of a major interruption to normal activity. Ideally, a plan of action should exist which will ensure seamless recovery from a disaster.

History and background

Disaster recovery

When computers were first introduced, as a means for storing and manipulating data, it quickly became apparent that organisations and individuals needed to be able to recover their work when a machine became unstable and the saved data was corrupted. This process became known as disaster recovery or DR. The technique became familiar to IT professionals but remained little understood by general management.

Business recovery

With the passage of time and the introduction of distributed systems via servers and networks, and latterly personal computers, it soon became clear that information systems are an integral support function to organisations, rather than separate systems in their own right. Managers began to consider investing in broader disaster recovery contingency plans. However, they soon realised that if a disaster happened – say, a major fire in a production area – the fact that the computer could be restored while the work accommodation for staff could not, seemed a little like putting the cart before the horse. From this developed the term 'business recovery' which involved not just computer systems but business processes and human interaction more broadly.

Maintaining business as usual

Since the introduction of the computer age, the speed of service delivery has increased and the concept of business recovery has been found in practice to be too little too late. It is not sufficient to simply recover from a disaster, as during which time competitors and/or customers may have lost patience and moved their business elsewhere. Instead, it is now necessary to examine how to maintain business as usual. For this new situation, the term 'business continuity' is used to cover the strategic vision of an organisation and maintain its customer service.

In the service and healthcare sector, the prospect of clients moving to a competitor does not exist in quite the same way as in commercial organisations, although doubtless any major impact to service delivery will influence referral patterns and purchase of services. Instead, we frequently observe a public which is increasingly less tolerant of service delays or interruption and which measures an organisation's reputation and its public face by how well the organisation manages its continuous operation.

The need to have contingency plans in place has been recognised for some time in larger hospitals, and many initiatives have been tried and tested. It is possible to develop simple but effective service continuity plans. The basis for successful planning is executive sponsorship and adoption of a top-down approach. This means planning for impact mitigation, rather than for every possible eventuality.

What is service continuity management?

The use of the phrase 'service continuity management' is deliberate. It is a management process and it needs to be championed from the top of an organisation. Often the term continuity planning is used, but this is only one part of the process of managing the service continuity of the organisation. Circumstances, procedures and staff changes mean that the process must be ongoing, with a regular schedule of review and update. Essentially, management must strive for a constant state of preparedness at all levels.

For service continuity management to be effective, a strategic decision must be made at executive level to put in place an action plan. This must be robust and comprehensive enough to ensure the continuity of core services even in the event of a major incident. It is not just about putting a plan in place as part of a new initiative; it must be recognised as part of the risk management process of ongoing mitigation and preparedness. It must be seen as a change to the way things are done.

Defining a 'major incident'

Part of the plan-building process requires the term 'major incident' to be defined. Such a definition can be based upon the existing definition contained within the major incident plan (MIP) of larger hospitals for external incidents, such as civil emergencies or road traffic accidents. The service continuity plan is, however, concerned with internal incidents. These incidents may or may not be equal in size to the external incident addressed by the MIP, but they do have very real impacts upon the organisation in terms of resolving the hazard or problem and managing the issues and implications arising from the incident. To be successful, it is necessary to prioritise and categorise activities within the organisation and determine each function's tolerance to interruption, in terms of:

- impact on interdependencies up-stream (who supplies us) and down-stream (who critically depends on us)

- scale – that is, minimum post-loss resource requirements for staff, accommodation, equipment, networks and communications

- duration (hours, days, weeks or longer)

Usually a major internal incident can be defined in terms of:

- preventing more than one function from continuing with its normal operations as a result of a genuine threat to life, facilities, utilities, and equipment, and

- falling outside the scope of normal management arrangements, with the potential to materially affect the activities or reputation of the organisation

Threats to service continuity

There are many threats impacting on a healthcare organisation's ability to deliver its services and serve the community. These can have an impact on both clinical and non-clinical areas (see box).

Potential threats

- fire or explosion affecting a department or centralised energy centre

- severe weather leading to flooding or burst pipes

- theft of care equipment

- hacking leading to breaches of data protection legislation and security of patient records

- supply chain failure in domestic or hotel services

- IT system failure blocking access to patient administration systems

- sub-standard performance in hygiene, catering, or clinical care

- infrastructure interruption, such as loss of utilities, medical gas supply or voice and data communication

---

To both multi-sited NHS trusts and single site healthcare providers, a major fire is an expensive and inconvenient interruption, with the potential to harm patients and staff as well as service delivery. The impact is not determined by the cause, but rather the effect on the organisation's service delivery. For example, consider the loss, by fire, to a hospital, of four medical wards versus loss of the centralised laundry.

Which has the larger impact? By contrast, the local ambulance station providing a 24-hour service to a number of client trusts would find it almost impossible to operate if the manufacturer of its fleet recommended a recall on safety grounds.

So we see that the impact of a major incident varies from one organisation to another. The philosophy of service continuity management is geared towards reducing the impact of interruption to a specific service by restoring its critical function, irrespective of the nature of the disaster.

Potential impact of incidents

For NHS organisations, potential impact really boils down to loss of service provision to any client group in the community. It is the standard of front-line services as judged by the public that sets the pace for continuity. Often, back-office support and management are not immediately critical.

Many organisations have failed to implement a service continuity culture simply by making a fundamental error – that is, misjudging what needs to be planned for. Many organisations recognise the need to conduct risk assessments, and in the process anticipate a considerable range of potential eventualities. An immediate response to this is often to seek to develop a contingency arrangement for each and every risk. This is simply an impossible task, as in any organisation there are many interdependencies and possibilities. Much time and resource will be expended attempting to come up with practical solutions that avoid the creation of other problems. A tactical solution or fix must be matched by an equally robust strategic consideration of the issues arising from any proposed solution.

Inability to provide a service is the worst case scenario and can be encapsulated in terms of loss of premises, systems, staff and equipment. This is what has to be planned for. If the impact of an event is not as serious as this, an organisation will be able to continue to use the services that remain to best effect.

How incidents are managed, and seen to be managed, can have a significant impact on an organisation's reputation and its ability to recover in the eyes of the community. A post-incident communication strategy is therefore a sensible measure.

The nature of disasters in healthcare

Some would argue that our working life is a constant series of crises or disasters – but this is not the case. It is the out-of-the-ordinary event that must be considered in service continuity planning.

Crises do not need to become disasters if they are managed correctly. Often in the healthcare sector, crisis communication is as important as crisis management. The news media will always pick up on a human story, such as:

* patient records found at the public refuse centre
* body parts found on a landfill site
* failure of management control over radiation doses for radiotherapy
* collapse of a patient record archive and library system
* failure of life support systems
* newly installed kitchens failing to meet food hygiene requirements

Mercifully the application of fire regulations in hospitals has resulted in very few catastrophic incidents relating to fire, so it is more worthwhile to look at other risks.

Causes of disaster

Disaster stories in the healthcare sector tend to focus on the organisation's treatment of a group of individuals. The Department of Health's report *An Organisation with a Memory* (see KEY REFERENCES, piii) states that incidents in trusts can be attributed to:

* 92% – lack of communication and systems
* 8% – human error

However, in reality most incidents are simply blamed on human error rather than recognising that the system might need to be reviewed. Systems should be in place to minimise the risk of error in human activity and in electro-mechanical devices.

If we consider near-misses or behaviour that could lead to a disaster, in light of the above, an example at a newly completed hospital with an adjacent energy centre proves the case in point (see box opposite).

We see in this example that a procedure not only needs to be documented, but also applied and enforced. A change in the cultural attitude to risk management is required. All parties in an organisation, whether public or private sector partners, must adopt an integrated approach. This is precisely the intended outcome from applying the 19 standards in the NHS controls assurance programme (see KEY REFERENCES, piii).

Jamming the door

The energy centre is in a separate, secure compound area at a major hospital, with an emergency exit door giving direct access to the main street. Inside the building are all the controls and plant to provide the hospital with standby power generation, day-to-day heating, ventilation and air conditioning.

The safe operation of the centre is placed with a service contractor subject to the professional controls expected for such a facility, including swipe card access control. Employees of the service contractor were formerly NHS trust staff and have close relations with trust staff employed in hotel duties. For ease of access to local shops, non-authorised trust personnel had bypassed the access control system with cooperation from contracted operating staff. Using the energy centre as a short cut, they had jammed the final exit door ajar so as to make their way to and from the hospital, instead of using the main entrance and road management system, which was a longer route.

This is not an isolated example but it highlights the potential for self-inflicted interruptions to occur. The risk of idle fingers touching controls they should not touch, in addition to individuals placing themselves in a compromised safety position, all points to a failure to appreciate the part everyone plays in maintaining a reduced risk environment.

Closure or interruption

Other examples of service interruption that should require the invocation of a coordinated response through the service continuity plan may include temporary closure of a maternity unit, or the accident and emergency unit or perhaps simultaneous failure of a number of life support systems. The duration of closure or interruption is one of the factors to consider when considering the impact and therefore the appropriateness of any contingency arrangement.

Incident creep

Without embarking on a prescriptive policy, it is useful for staff to have an aide-memoire setting out in broad terms what may be considered as a minor incident in order to differentiate it from a major incident. It is also important to get across the fact that incident creep can be a real issue – a minor incident without adequate response and control can become a major incident which eventually becomes much more difficult to control. So while demarcation between levels of incident can be useful, the cardinal rule with incident management, regardless of scale, is to attempt to gain control as soon as possible. Better to put in place a team to manage early, only to find that the situation can be addressed by line management, than to have senior management wishing they had put a team together a few hours previously.

Central coordination

Ideally, central coordination of what might be termed 'issues management' needs to be established. Locally, a manager may be unaware that while they are dealing with a major issue, others in the organisation may be dealing with similar or equally serious matters. Could it be that if the incidents are considered together, the service continuity plan should be put on standby or brought into play? Someone needs to be aware of all incidents and to manage service continuity from this holistic angle. It is best to encourage management to have local contingency arrangements for their service units, but when failure of the entire service unit is likely as a result of the incident, the service continuity plan should be invoked.

The impact of service interruption

Essentially, the impact of interruption on service delivery must be measured in terms of two components: scale and duration. In other words, every organisation has a tolerance level beyond which pain is experienced. In the health sector the pain is usually expressed in service downtime or patient complaint.

The scale of the interruption will range from affecting only one unit through to widespread disruption, and will depend on the delay before service can be resumed. The time period can have an impact in scale from inconvenient to life threatening.

Loss of facilities

Take the example of a complete failure of the centralised steam boiler. What impact will this have on a hospital's ability to function?

The absence of heating and hot water will be immediately critical for patients and staff and alternative arrangements will have to be made quickly. However, for some services – such as outpatients – it may be sufficient to arrange a local radio announcement indicating the intention to resume normal services in a few days' time.

Alternatively, consider control rooms and their communication facilities – can these be replicated off-site, or diverted to alternative facilities? Are there centralised environmental controls for heat, light, and water supplies? Should there be a sanctioned alternative arrangement?

What if an incident extends beyond 24 hours? Take fire or building asbestos contamination – will there be an exponential increase in the services affected?

Loss of staff

The questions posed above concern the physical environment, but the healthcare sector has no greater asset than its people. Contingency plans must consider the impact of loss of staff. Annual influenza outbreaks affect not just the public but also staff. A major accident involving serious loss of life can have very traumatic consequences and requires a unique sensitivity. Organisations should ensure that service continuity plans include plans to cope with reduced staffing levels, and post-incident management and communication.

Resources

The larger the concern over the business impact, the greater the resources needed to cope with the consequences will be. Resources are not only financial – more often than not, it is about having the right people in the right place at the right time. The speed of attendance may be a key factor but so is competency – and it all comes back to preparedness. A suitable level of preparedness involves training in substitute equipment and methods of working. Clearly not all potential incidents present a common impact and therefore the level of resources and urgency of response for each will vary.

Getting the balance right is difficult, but it is a decision that must be made, periodically reviewed and adjusted by senior management. Often it is a judgment call because not all major incidents clearly manifest their implications immediately. A fire or major building failure may be the exception.

With careful thought, it is not difficult to imagine the impact of a major incident, yet it is not something that many in senior management seem to consider without being prompted during a service continuity management project.

Business impact: strategic principles

Why not consider what a disaster would mean, in the cool light of day? A number of strategic principles need to be considered:

- Can the organisation prioritise its response to an incident?

- Are some services more critical than others?

- Which services would the organisation defend at all costs?

- What are the factors influencing such a selection of priorities?

- What are the political, reputational, geographical, financial and demographic influences?

- Who might need to know about an incident?

- What would the organisation say in defence of its actions?

- What might be the consequences of such a statement?

- Who else will be involved?

- Who would the organisation want to involve?

- Who does the organisation want to make sure is not involved?

This thought process can form the basis for considering a management strategy. This strategy needs to be clear about the recovery objective. If the objective is known it is much easier to focus on achieving an agreed course of management action.

The next step is to convey the strategy to staff at all levels. They need to make a commitment to mitigation activity from identified threats, agree the appropriate level of preparedness and have confidence in organisation-wide and departmental service continuity plans to reduce the impact of an interruption.

Developing service continuity plans

Under the direction of hospital accident and emergency units, major incident plans have been in place for many years, to cope professionally and sensitively with disasters. These plans sit alongside local authorities' generic emergency plans involving the emergency services, social services and other statutory and voluntary organisations.

Such plans are intended to cope, for example, with a weather event, a community calamity, an explosion or a transport accident. Depending upon the degree of involvement and professional expertise required, some plans require more detail than others. In the same way, NHS trusts need to develop a range of internal action plans to ensure continuity of service.

Internal action plans

Internal action plans are based on the premise that continuity of service provision to the local community is a prerequisite, not least because:

- the population's tolerance of service interruption is ever-diminishing

- maintenance of the trust or service provider's reputation, in the eyes of the public and the health authority, is essential

- the chief executive has to satisfy elected representatives and trust boards that in the event of an emergency all is being done that can be done

Three phases of response

A clearly thought out and predetermined action plan involving all staff at all levels needs to be implemented, including the strategic response of senior management in a crisis management plan, as well as a detailed functional or tactical response of departmental staff in their service recovery plan. By breaking the evolution of the incident down into three defined phases (see Figure 1 overleaf) it is possible to allocate responsibilities and inform staff where they fit in.

The people involved

Before embarking on a service continuity project it is essential to ensure the project has the sponsorship of the chief executive, or most

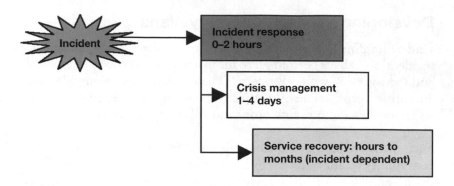

Figure 1: Three phases of response

senior manager, and that the project is not seen as yet another initiative over which heads of directorates and departments can prioritise their attention. In today's working environment there is real danger in project overload. It is therefore essential that the project is monitored at the highest level and those involved are supported.

When developing functional service continuity plans it is important to have directorate and department heads on board throughout, and to this end, it is prudent to have a project steering group. This should include the senior management team, since they already have a firm grasp of the organisation's strategic direction and its key responsibilities in an external incident. It can be useful to demonstrate that external major accident plans can be used as a basis, subject to modification, for the creation of internal service continuity plans.

Keep it simple

For a plan to work, it must be simple and easy to use. A complete version will be held by the plan coordinator and team leaders, but individual members of the teams, with specific responsibilities, need only have, for example, their actions recorded on a laminated A4 card.

It must be remembered that the plan will be used in a stressful situation by individuals, each of whom will bring to the event their own frame of mind and level of competence. This should be borne in mind when selecting the language and phraseology used in the plan. It must reflect the culture and terminology of the organisation and not introduce a new vocabulary.

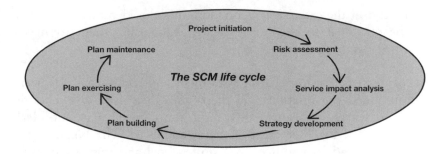

Figure 2: The service continuity management life cycle

Life cycle

Typically service continuity management should establish and then repeat a life cycle of phased activities. First, the steering group must decide where in the life cycle it considers the organisation to be in the development of its service continuity management culture. The lifecycle can be graphically shown as depicted in Figure 2.

Project initiation

This first stage of a service continuity programme involves obtaining commitment from senior management and project personnel to agree the scope, objectives, method, timing, work schedule and budget. It also examines the existing tolerance to interruption in different aspects of the organisation, and produces an incident definition and high-level incident management command and control structure.

Risk assessment

Organisations adopting the NHS controls assurance standards (see p222) will be familiar with the development of a risk register. Integral to the process must be an element of risk assessment. This is the basis on which all of the organisation's risks are identified, evaluated and given a score or ranking in terms of impact and likelihood. The exercise facilitates a mechanism to manage risk in the organisation across a whole range of issues, typically grouped into three risk categories:

- **strategic risk** – reputation, service offering, political direction
- **operational risk** – personnel, health and safety, property assets, healthcare procedures
- **financial risk** – budget controls, contract terms

At the end of the exercise a report outlining the identified risk areas can be presented to the board which will enable them to make informed loss mitigation choices.

Frequently, where a formal risk assessment and register has not been commissioned, organisations will cherry-pick their risks for attention, based on whatever is apparently most pressing. This is not ideal because underlying root causes are not addressed. The board really ought to expend its resources in a professional and transparent way consistent with corporate governance and controls assurance. To do this a full register of risks is required.

The risk assessment process is a useful prelude to the service continuity process because it can point to the major risks that should be considered in the impact analysis stage. There is one proviso, however: when considering interruption to services the concept of probability or likelihood is unhelpful. A risk may be classified as a one in a 100-year event, but what if it occurred tomorrow?

A risk register should be used for base information, but the impact of loss should be reconsidered in the service impact analysis (SIA) stage.

Service impact analysis

The SIA considers the critical processes in an organisation and assesses the impact of the risks identified in the risk assessment. Essentially it is about listing all that is done under normal conditions.

Each process is considered in relation to all other functions, and then prioritised in order of recovery to minimise the damage to service continuity in the event of an incident. In addition, upstream and downstream interdependencies, mitigation or protection arrangements, and the current state of preparedness, if any, for recovery are examined.

Recovery options must be considered, minimum post-loss resource requirements identified, and recovery milestones along a timeline introduced.

Recovery strategy

Agreeing a service continuity strategy is only the first step. In order to implement it, financial and staff resources will be necessary. Certain items might need to be purchased, installed and linked to existing processes. Contracts might need to be entered into with third parties, or other arrangements put in place, such as mutual aid or reciprocal agreements.

Staff will probably require training, given that for some the handling of an emergency situation will be alien to their usual day job. Certainly, work around methods for current practice will need to be agreed – such as alternative procedures to resuscitate a hospital patient should the defibrillators malfunction simultaneously.

The formation of a service continuity strategy demonstrates the security of the organisation's critical processes to community stakeholders. It also gives the senior management group an opportunity to benchmark their recovery strategies against healthcare standards.

Plan writing

The plan will be used by ordinary people at all organisational levels and must, therefore, be easily comprehensible. One moment they may be operating in normal conditions, the next potentially in chaos. The plan should be snappy and easy to use. In the first instance, the concern is to learn the facts – the what, why, where, when, and who. Those called upon to react can often be faced with sensory overload. Why not establish the communication channels in advance and determine who needs to know and when?

Five requirements of a sound plan

On the basis of a sound command and control structure, a plan can be condensed into five main sections:

- corporate policy and incident command and control

- emergency response in the first hours following an incident

- crisis management in the first days following an incident

- service recovery from day one until the full recovery of the organisation

- contact details listing who needs to be told and where assistance is to be sought

Corporate policy and incident command and control

The introduction to the plan must contain minimal detail. Users of a plan should be familiar with the history of the plan's development; while the plan coordinator will have good reason to detail a background and plan maintenance records, these are not required in an incident and can be placed in an alternative document. What is needed here is a quick reminder of how the plan will work and who will be responsible for what action.

Emergency response in the first hours following an incident

This element of the plan is location-specific and forms a tactical response to an immediate situation. It could be a physical event such as loss of power or accommodation, but equally it could be an IT failure, or perhaps a serious complaint with the potential for impact on an organisation's reputation. The team involved in emergency response should be drawn from across the organisation and may co-opt assistance beyond the team as the occasion dictates.

Crisis management in the first days following an incident

This is the strategic response to a report of an incident coming from the emergency response team, which should comprise the senior management team. Their objective must be to be able to pull back from the immediate response activity and consider strategic issues and implications. Where does this situation place the organisation in terms of its responsibilities and its vision statement? In the light of this requirement the team needs to establish a command centre as the hub of management activity.

The most critical aspect of their work is communication to all the stakeholders in the community and in the organisation itself. It is from the command centre that press and media response should be coordinated. The strategic direction and the pre-agreed recovery strategies will require regular review and, potentially, modification in light of the situation as it evolves. Ultimately return to a position of some normality is needed even if it means working from temporary accommodation within a week.

Interestingly, the impact of a disaster or major incident can be the first occasion when the calibre of the management team is actually observed by an external constituency. It is therefore essential for the preservation of the organisation and the directors to be seen to be able to handle such an event competently. Media training is a prerequisite.

Service recovery from day one until the full recovery of the organisation

This element of the service continuity plan is crucial. Using a generic template, filling in the boxes without understanding the need, is a recipe for failure. Building upon the foundation work done in the service impact analysis, alternative arrangements to deliver continuity of service can be recorded for each of the organisation's functions.

Clearly where a major interruption has occurred, access may be denied to accommodation or staff are unable to fulfil their roles, it will be impossible to restore all functions simultaneously. That is why it is important to rank the order of recovery in terms of priority. In addition, an understanding of knock-on effects can be gleaned from an interdependency study.

At the end of the exercise each directorate or department should have their own version of the plan, specific to their area. A composite plan will be held at the command centre and by the plan coordinator.

Contact details listing who needs to be told and where assistance is to be sought

A comprehensive database of contacts must be developed. Not surprisingly, this is the one element of the plan, which is constantly changing and should be regularly reviewed.

Plans often focus on the specific recovery of critical service provision. Each section of the plan must consider who is involved, their roles, responsibilities and what action is likely to be needed, how this is to be carried out and in what order. The plan needs to be flexible and action-oriented. Planning for the worst eventuality – typically a denied access situation – means the plan will meet the needs of any situation.

Plan exercising

To write a plan is only the first step. Few plans in their first appearance are fully satisfactory.

It is essential to prove to the teams that what has been written will meet the objectives of recovery and service continuity. The use of the term 'exercising' is deliberate. It is not about testing or giving marks out of 10. It is about rehearsing the people through their action steps and giving them experience of working in an out-of-the-ordinary situation and one which is potentially very stressful.

Plan exercising can range from a talk through to full simulation, including evacuation of the site, full exercise of the plan and media exposure of senior management.

Component-level exercising

Exercising should be done in component level to start with; it is never wise to try and do a full simulation of the whole plan as a first event. It is necessary to build up competence levels in all the teams and sort out the apparent difficulties of each before bringing them together.

One component, which is easy to do, and will reveal any communication weaknesses in the plan, is to exercise the call cascade or contact list in the plan. On the basis of those individuals able to respond to a phone call over a weekend, for example, you can determine how easily the plan could be implemented. Many plans have failed at the first hurdle because the phone number is not correct or there is no out-of-hours contact number.

Plan exercising identifies the improvement areas required in the plan, and provides hands-on experience for all staff involved. It validates the work done to date and, if done correctly, will ensure that no team or group of individuals is more advanced in their state of preparedness than others.

Plan maintenance

The maintenance of the service continuity plan is as crucial as its development. Nobody writes an operating performance plan for one financial year to have it gather dust in the next. It is constantly reviewed and updated in the light of the operating environment. The same must apply to a service continuity plan. Ideally managers should see its maintenance as part of their responsibilities consistent with the controls assurance programme.

If exercising is done on a regular basis (at least annually) then it can be expected that the plan will automatically require updating and refining. Certainly managers should be encouraged to review their plan biannually looking, in particular, to ensure the document reflects the current service offering, since in some instances this may have changed since the plan was first written.

Implementation of service continuity plans

The vision at all times is of a plan that is easily usable by all levels in an organisation, even under adverse conditions. Staff will not want to use large lever-arch file plans, which are heavy in descriptive text, under such circumstances.

As previously discussed, the plans can be structured under the headings of emergency response, crisis management and service recovery. This gives the senior management team a clear picture.

Implementation of a service continuity plan is initially resource-hungry, until such time as it can be signed off, subject to modification through rehearsal and exercising. Like any project that is worth doing, management and staff should be clear on the deliverables and timescale to achieve them.

Sometimes there can be objections to putting these resources together. In addition, there may be a cost implication. The use of external resources to assist the project, lend it weight and deliver a tried and tested methodology can be seen as a cost. A more positive perspective would be to see it as an investment.

External assistance

External assistance can be very useful and usually comes in two forms: consultancy and software.

Consultancy

Engaging a consultant should be done after examining their credentials. A track record in service continuity should be expected, and previous experience in the healthcare sector would be useful. It is worth enquiring as to their adherence to the 10 standards advocated by the Business Continuity Institute (see p223).

Their competency must be ascertained. Do they come with a technical or information systems bias or a wider organisational focus? Remember the subtle distinction between disaster recovery of the IT system as distinct from service continuity management of the whole organisation.

There is no doubt that a consultant will bring to the organisation a tried and tested methodology, which, with careful agreement with the organisation's plan coordinator, should minimise the amount of management input required, whilst maintaining sufficient ownership. Some consultancies will encourage the use of bespoke planning software while others prefer using the office packages in common use. There is no hard and fast rule.

Software

Software can be useful, particularly where an internal plan coordinator has limited experience and is quite keen on an IT solution. There are, however, some drawbacks. What you get is what you see. These are off-the-shelf packages and customisation will be down to the user. It will be up to the user to use whatever parts of the software they deem appropriate. If they are not entirely sure what they want to achieve, there is a danger that a fill-in-the-box approach may be adopted without due care, resulting in critical parts of a plan being omitted.

Complex inter-relationship databases can be very clever, but it does rather lock the plan coordinator into being the author, editor and reviser for all future versions of the plan. This could be quite a workload and reduces the opportunity for sharing ownership of the planning process.

Ideally, the plan coordinator wants to engage the whole organisation and therefore present the plan in a format that is familiar to the end user. This leads to a coordination management role enabling a more holistic approach to training, exercising, maintenance and auditing programmes.

Rebutting objections

Regardless of the approach adopted, there are bound to be objections from some quarters. It might therefore be helpful to present some of the arguments here and suggest some rebuttals:

We can't afford it/we don't need it

Can your organisation afford to be without a service continuity plan? Research has shown that effective continuity management greatly reduces post-disaster losses. It also brings additional advantage in encouraging a broader risk management culture.

It requires too much management time

Management involvement is essential to ensure proper ownership of the project and delivery to schedule. Ideally, the project coordinator should look to spread the load across the organisation.

We've done disaster recovery

Service continuity management is more than disaster recovery. Disaster recovery is focused upon IT, whereas service continuity management looks across the whole of the organisation.

We already have a plan

Has it been exercised or audited? Would it stand up to a benchmark review? Can you be sure the format is suitable for use in a crisis? If you have any doubts about your existing plan, now is the time to engage a review before it is found wanting in a real and stressful situation.

Putting service continuity plans into practice

It is often stated that a plan must be a living document. The core ingredient of any workable plan is a robust and comprehensive command, control and communication protocol. Plans should be action-oriented, yet strategic, looking across the whole of the organisation, while usable at working level within individual departments. They should be focused upon loss of key functional ability from whatever cause, rather than being related to specific incidents. Ideally, the team which builds the plan will be the team called upon to implement it in the event of a real incident.

So where does the theory meet with the practice? A plan lying on the shelf in a director's office is no use – it just gathers dust. What is required is a programme of training and rehearsal that reduces the unknown element and surprise often experienced by those with little or no previous experience. One team gaining experience at the expense of others in the organisation is also counter-productive.

Plan components

As demonstrated in this chapter, the service continuity plan is actually a group of plans. Each can be seen as a component of the whole. Circumstances may dictate that it is appropriate in certain instances to use one component at a time, for example, to bring the crisis management team together for a significant event, however generally they are interrelated.

It is important to recognise the component nature of the plan in relation to the principal teams, that is:

- emergency response
- crisis management
- departmental recovery

Training

The next step is to train each team in its role and clearly amplify their responsibilities as detailed in the plan.

Figure 4 shows the effectiveness of a service continuity training programme that will raise the levels of competence equally across the organisation. While it could be argued that some training is better than none, the left chart is not as effective as the right.

Effective training needs to be imaginative but realistic. There is little point in the UK of running a scenario involving an earthquake or tornado. People like to have a reference point, so a realistic scenario perhaps involving the breakdown of the central laundry, kitchen or energy centre is a good starting point.

Preparedness

Who will be the first to recognise an incident? What should be their reaction? Does the plan detail who should be informed and when? What will the informed person's reaction be?

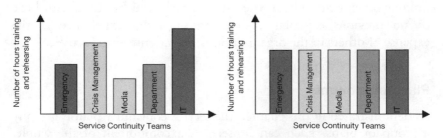

Figure 4: Levels of training in different teams

Preparedness

In the emergency team it is a good idea to revolve the first on the call-out list. This enables more than a few to experience the leadership required in the plan. That way holidays, illness and attendance at conferences can be covered. Essentially the revolving role of leader in both the emergency and crisis team can be equated to the passing of the baton in a relay race.

By developing the scenario other facets of the plan will be highlighted. Who in the organisation is good at media handling? Is further training needed from specialists in this area? Will the timeline on the recovery of the IT systems and applications marry with the end user requirements and their recovery timeline?

By encouraging a culture of training and preparedness within the organisation, there is no doubt the teams will be able to handle the unexpected competently and robustly. Not only that, they will have tangible proof of their compliance with the controls assurance programme which can in turn be demonstrated to their local stakeholders.

A strategic investment

Any successful modern organisation strives to achieve optimum service through a combination of the right strategy and maximisation of its resources. We have seen this in the healthcare sector:

- corporate restructuring – creation, merging and de-merging of trusts
- aggressive strategies to address increased utilisation of staff and mission-critical resources
- commercial integration or partnership with third-party suppliers
- implementation of just-in-time processes
- a focus on quality as well as value
- compliance with governance programmes, sector regulations and requirements
- changes in strategic direction or the introduction of new services
- complex interdependencies and a growing reliance on third parties in the delivery of service

- increased communication with more demanding stakeholders

Critical to the success of many of these initiatives is good project management, and integral to the project management approach must be a recognition of the part played by risk management in general and service continuity in particular. Service continuity management is a vital component in the delivery of these strategies, as well as a key discipline in the successful day-to-day management of any organisation. Service continuity strategies must link directly with what matters in delivering a level of service to the public.

For an organisation valuing its people, running critical IT and facilities, and investing in its reputation and community perception, service continuity represents a comparatively small investment in exchange for operational security and peace of mind.

In an increasingly intolerant world, a successful service continuity programme is often a source of distinct reputational advantage. The alternative is an unprepared organisation displaying its inefficiencies in an unsuccessfully managed interruption.

Service continuity management as part of the holistic risk management programme must be seen as a strategic investment, not a cost, involving all layers within the organisation.

NHS Executive controls assurance standards – non-clinical

1. Risk management system
2. Buildings, land plant, and non-medical equipment
3. Catering and food hygiene
4. Contracts and control of contractors
5. Emergency preparedness
6. Environmental management
7. Fire safety
8. Health and safety management
9. Human resources
10. Infection control
11. Information management and technology
12. Medical devices management
13. Medicines management

14. Professional and product liability
15. Records management
16. Security
17. Transport
18. Waste management
19. De-contamination

Ten standards of the Business Continuity Institute

1. Project initiation and management
2. Risk evaluation and control
3. Business impact analysis
4. Developing business continuity strategies
5. Emergency response and operations
6. Developing and implementing business continuity plans
7. Awareness and training programmes
8. Maintaining and exercising business continuity plans
9. Public relations and crisis coordination
10. Coordination with public authorities

Useful websites

- Business Continuity Institute: *www.thebci.com*
- Government Emergency Planning Division: *www.homeoffice.gov.uk/epd*
- Survive (membership group for business continuity professionals): *www.survive.com*

Online services

- Crisis navigator (internet guide to crisis management): *www.crisisnavigator.org*
- *www.disasterplan.com*
- Emergencynet (online emergency news and analysis): *www.emergency.com*
- Globalcontinuity.com (information on business risk and continuity planning): *www.globalcontinuity.com*

Courses and literature:

- Glasgow Caledonian University: *www.gcal.ac.uk*

- Rothstein Associates Inc (book and software catalogue): *www.rothstein.com*
- Scarman Centre at the University of Leicester: *www.le.ac.uk/scarman/cp.html*
- University of Sheffield: *www.shef.ac.uk*

9 Managing people

Janet Martin

This chapter covers:

- **Workforce expansion**
- **Lessons from high-profile reports**
- **Recruitment and selection procedures**
- **Induction training, appraisal and revalidation**
- **Leadership and management training**
- **Staff retention and morale**
- **The statutory framework**

Chapter 2 defines risk management and the strategies for managing risk as part of organisational processes. It shows how risk management is a learning process and how organisations must understand the causes of risk in order to then introduce proper control measures. The links with quality and high standards of care provision are also explored.

Managing change

The organisation of healthcare in the UK is undergoing great change: the introduction of primary care and mental health trusts, and strategic health authorities being obvious examples. Whenever change is planned, the human resource management priority is to identify the issues, by which we generally mean the constraints and the risks. The risks are those arising from not getting it right, both in terms of statutory requirements (for example, consultation and employee transfers), but also in managing the people affected by the change to ensure the continuing effective and safe delivery of services.

People management processes

Similarly, from the point of view of the daily running of health services, there are issues, or risks, arising from people management processes. Processes affecting an employee's journey through an organisation, from recruitment and induction, through appraisal and development, to termination arrangements, can lead to risks if not carried out effectively.

This chapter aims to explore this journey, and to examine how risks can arise at different stages, the potential impact on employee behaviour and on the organisation and successful healthcare delivery. It also aims to address the human resource solutions to these risks, and to offer practical advice to managers in handling the situations and risks which can arise when managing people.

The link between staff and service

The point has already been made that risk management spans all functions in the organisation. This chapter also aims to show how effective people management underpins the reduction of risk in healthcare and links into clinical governance and improving the quality of care for patients. One of the core principles embodied in the NHS Plan (see KEY REFERENCES, piii) is the need to work continuously to improve health services and to minimise errors. The link between high-quality staff, quality services and reducing errors is a major theme of current thinking, carried forward into the national goal for every healthcare organisation to be a model employer through good human resource management.

Workforce expansion

Investment in staff

The NHS Plan announced expansion in staff numbers by 2004, comprising 20,000 more nurses, 7,500 more consultants, 2,000 more GPs and 6,500 more therapists and other health professionals, to meet its overall goals for achieving improvements in the quality of healthcare. However, the follow up report, *Investment and reform for NHS Staff – taking forward the NHS Plan*[1] recognises that recruitment is not the only issue. There needs to be investment in staff in order to produce a quality workforce. This means modernising professional education and training, and introducing family-friendly employment policies to ensure that scarce healthcare skills and expertise are not lost.

Restoring public confidence

Underlying all this is the need to restore public confidence in the delivery of healthcare. High-profile reports on events at Bristol Royal Infirmary (see KEY REFERENCES, piii) and the Royal Liverpool Children's Hospital have identified a raft of failings. Similarly, the Clothier and Bullock reports (analysed below) into the issues arising from the activities of individual health workers, and other reports concerning GP and locum appointments, have raised deep criticisms of traditional practice. Although these reports relate to clinical staff, the problems identified, and the action to raise standards are equally applicable to other healthcare workers.

There are human resource management solutions to many of the risks identified in the reports, including recommendations on recruitment, selection, training, appraisal, supervision and leadership. It is important to learn from these experiences, and incorporate their lessons into strategies for good employment practice for all healthcare workers, in order to manage the risks arising from individual behaviour or organisational failings.

Lessons from Allitt and others

Over the last 10 years there have been a number of incidents where the actions of individuals have resulted in patient harm and public concern about the safety of care. These all have lessons for human resource practitioners in the same way as they have for other healthcare managers and professionals.

The report of the inquiry into the case of enrolled nurse Beverley Allitt[2] describes how during early 1991 there was a series of incidents on the children's ward at Grantham Hospital. Three children died suddenly on the ward, and one at home not long after discharge. Nine other children collapsed unexpectedly, some more than once.

In many of the cases it seemed to the doctors on the ward that what had happened was unusual, but could be explained on the basis of the children's medical history. Nevertheless, suspicion grew that these might be cases of deliberate harm. A police investigation took place, and Beverley Allitt was charged with four murders and nine attempted murders.

The Clothier report

The Clothier report into the case was critical of both senior management in the hospital, and nurse management on the ward for failing to act when suspicions first arose.

Criticisms

The report also found the background to the employment of Beverley Allitt as an enrolled nurse was "unsatisfactory". She had an exceptionally high level of sickness as a student nurse, missing 126 days during the nurse-training course, and was later found to display evidence of a major personality disorder. Yet her health record was disregarded, and referral for assessment by the occupational health department was neglected.

The managerial procedures for the appointment itself were described as "sloppy". There were no records of an application form being completed, and no written references. The personnel department was not informed of her appointment, and there were delays in issuing a contract of employment. Beverley Allitt had started work before any health screening took place, and despite the requirement for managers to check that a candidate has no previous criminal convictions before appointment to a post with substantial access to children, no police check was made. In fact she had no previous convictions, but the inquiry found the failure to follow normal procedures "extremely worrying".

Recommendations

The recommendations of the inquiry included the following on nurse appointments:

- In addition to routine references, the most recent employer or place of study should be asked to provide at least a record of time taken off on grounds of sickness.

- No candidate for nursing in whom there is evidence of major personality disorder should be employed in the profession.

- Nurses should undergo formal health screening when they obtain their first posts after qualifying.

The case of Beverley Allitt is an extreme one, and the report acknowledges: "No measures can afford complete protection against a determined miscreant. The main lesson from the inquiry, and our principle recommendation, is that the Grantham disaster should serve to heighten awareness in all those caring for children of the possibility of malevolent intervention as a cause of unexpected critical events." The case is a good example of how low-risk probability can have a high impact in terms of consequences to patient care and damage to public confidence. This is also seen in the following reports.

The Bullock report

This report[3] looked at the case of Amanda Jenkinson, who was employed as a nurse in the intensive therapy unit at Bassetlaw District General Hospital, and in January 1994 was alleged to have tampered with equipment on the unit, putting patients at risk. She was suspended from duty and a series of investigations took place extending over several years. These resulted in a police prosecution, a conviction for serious assault and a prison sentence.

Failure to report medical history

Amanda Jenkinson was dismissed by the trust in 1995, not for any action while on the intensive therapy unit, but for an alleged failure to report fully her medical history. The report of the independent inquiry set up by North Nottinghamshire Health Authority states: "A determined and devious deceiver will always be difficult to detect, but a series of nets to catch such an employee or recruit could be constructed by means of cross-checking information from the applicant against that given by previous employers, occupational health departments and the employee's GP."

The report notes that although the hospital obtained references from previous employers, they were let down by the nature of the references which, seen retrospectively, were ambiguous and did not deal with the problems encountered by these previous employers. Taking references supplied to other trusts together, the report says, a pattern emerges of a character with difficulty accepting guidance, discipline or superior authority.

Recommendations

A number of recommendations are made on references, including that a standard form should be used, and that references should deal with fact rather than impressions. Where impressions are conveyed, factual examples or evidence should substantiate those impressions.

The report also recommends greater consistency in interview techniques and documentation, and the training of all those involved in the recruitment and selection process. A structured process with probing, relevant questions at interview would almost certainly have picked up the earlier concerns, and enabled them to be tested and verified.

General practice

Harold Shipman, a Manchester GP, was convicted in January 2000 of the murders of 15 elderly women in his care. A Department of Health audit of his career later found that he recorded 297 more deaths of patients than other doctors, 236 of which were at home. The outcome of the public inquiry is awaited, but selection and performance processes in general practice are already coming under scrutiny.

The Commission for Health Improvement (CHI) inquiry report into the case of Peter Green, a Loughborough GP jailed for eight years in July 2000 after being found guilty of abusing patients, says there must be a more open and honest system for appointing GPs. The introduction of standard systems for the appointment of GPs, whether as partners or single-handed practitioners, is more difficult because of their independent employment status. However, all appointments should follow the good practice processes outlined in this chapter, with proper checks made. Outside assessors should be involved to ensure independent, professional scrutiny and avoid the risk these cases highlight.

Employing locum consultants

The Elwood case

James Elwood was a retired consultant who worked as a short-term locum in several NHS hospitals. Concerns arose about discrepancies between his histopathology reports and the findings of other clinicians, but not before a number of patients had received inappropriate treatment as a result of errors in diagnosis, with serious consequences in seven cases.

The Secretary of State for Health asked CHI to investigate the use of locum medical practitioners in four NHS trusts, with particular reference to Dr Elwood. Its report[4] notes that the case has been the subject of considerable national and local publicity. It generated public and professional concern about medical errors and locum doctors. It also raises several important issues for the health service about the recruitment and management of doctors who move around the service, working for short periods in different places, and how concerns about clinical competence are communicated between employers.

Like others in England and Wales, the four trusts investigated by CHI make use of locum medical practitioners at various levels of seniority to cover holiday and study leave, unfilled posts, and to supplement staff at times of particular pressure. Appointments are usually needed at very short notice and for a relatively short time (days or weeks). There is a temptation not to be as thorough as for permanent appointments, but the risks, as the Elwood case shows, are just as great.

CHI report

The CHI report found that reliance on locum consultants is frequently due to poor workforce planning, particularly in terms of arrangements for covering leave for permanent consultants, and is often a substitute for the appointment of additional permanent consultants. In the field of histopathology, such problems are compounded by a shortage of qualified consultants.

Appointment

There is a DoH Code of Practice[5] on the appointment of locum doctors, but CHI found the four trusts concerned consistently failed to comply with these rules, and meet their duty of care to patients in employing doctors of proven ability to fulfil their responsibilities. The report describes how the trusts failed to use adequate safeguards when obtaining references, checking career history, interviewing, carrying out health checks and during induction.

Older doctors

The report also found that there were not enough safeguards in the employment of older doctors. The trusts complied with DoH guidance[6] on employing doctors over retirement age, and obtained the appropriate variation order. However, the national guidance does not require checks on the doctor's physical or mental ability to perform his duties – checks which were not done.

Performance monitoring

Performance monitoring of locum consultants was also poor, with little systematic checking of the quality or accuracy of their work.

CHI recommends that locums should be subject to the same system of clinical audit and performance monitoring as their permanent colleagues. There should be routine checking of locum consultants' work by an identified clinical supervisor and early notification of the medical director when errors or a pattern of poor practice are identified.

Communication between trusts

CHI also found a serious problem in ensuring that concerns about the performance or conduct of locum doctors are communicated between trusts and around the NHS generally. Too often the solution is to terminate employment, without advising other healthcare employers that there may be a risk. This is likely to be covered by new arrangements.

The Bristol inquiry (Kennedy report)

The risk outcome from an episode such as that at Bristol Royal Infirmary (see KEY REFERENCES, piii) is the consequential damage to the organisation's reputation and the professionals involved. The patient safety issues also have lessons for human resource practitioners.

The case

This was the largest ever investigation into clinical practice in the NHS, triggered by infant deaths during surgery in the late 1980s and early 1990s. Despite concerns about death rates raised by a whistleblower, by colleagues and by parents, surgeons at the Bristol Royal Infirmary failed to recognise or admit this, and continued to operate.

Culture

How did this happen? Culture has already been identified as a high-risk area for any organisation, and the inquiry report found too much arrogance, ambition and muddling through at the hospital, with a 'club culture' which shut out young doctors. A blame culture in particular contributed to senior doctors' refusal to recognise that mistakes were being made. The Health Secretary said: "If the NHS is to learn when things go wrong, it must move beyond a culture of blame." Introduction of audit and appraisal, discussed later, are key outcomes.

Skills

The report also cites the lack of requirement for consultants to keep their skills up to date. "Once qualified, the prevailing view was that it was up to them to maintain their competence save in exceptional circumstances... The hospital consultant effectively has a job for life."

Accountability

Accountability is a key issue in understanding the nature of risk. The relationship between clinicians and managers often focuses on volume of clinical activity, with too little concept of accountability to an employer; rather the concept of clinical freedom assumes doctors are accountable to their patients to obtain the best for them. Yet it is a reasonable assumption that the board of a trust should take steps to assess the risk to the public, and is responsible if the public is not adequately protected.

Further points

There are two other important points from the inquiry on the people agenda:

- The NHS must put patients at its core. They must be treated with respect – this requires a cultural, behavioural and attitude change.

- Care must be as safe as possible – requiring good recruitment and selection, appraisal and training, revalidation and continuing professional development.

The DoH's response in January 2002 summarises the action to be taken in detail.

The inquiry report also highlighted issues about teamworking and leadership. Poor teamwork had "implications for performance and outcome". The report says the relationship between the various professional groups was sometimes poor, demonstrating a lack of leadership. The medical director was described as having "power but no leadership".

Understaffing was also a factor, and this is developed further in the section on the need for adequate resources.

The Royal Liverpool inquiry

This inquiry[7] resulted from public concerns about the removal, retention, and disposal of human tissue and organs without proper consent or senior management knowledge of the extent of the practice. The report, published in January 2001, reiterates many issues about clinical governance covered in the Bristol inquiry. It also formulates management standards, three of which are relevant to people management, and are summarised in the recommendations as follows:

- No clinician should be appointed to a position of managerial authority in a hospital without having relevant clinical experience for the position.

- No clinician should take effective control of a management position until trained in all necessary management techniques and in any relevant legal requirements.

- Hospital managers should be of a suitable background and calibre for the role expected of them, provided with all the necessary training (including continued education) and themselves regularly appraised for the quality of their performance.

Major changes on consent are to be introduced; there will be training in organ retention and obtaining consent from relatives. Human resource managers have to ensure this training is incorporated into trust induction and other education programmes.

Summary of the lessons learnt

The human resource lessons learnt from these inquiries and reports are summarised in the table opposite. Many are recruitment issues, but others have a wider organisational context.

How these and other people management risk issues can be addressed, and used to enhance the value of people management to the business of the organisation, is examined in the remainder of the chapter.

Report/inquiry	Issues
Clothier report	References Occupational health involvement Interview technique Systems
Bullock report	References Occupational health involvement Interview process Recruitment and selection training
General practice	Appointment processes Fitness to practise
Use of locums	Recruitment References Career history Fitness to practise Alerting other employers Appraisal Identifying and learning from errors
Bristol Royal Infirmary (Kennedy report)	Culture Appraisal, revalidation and continuing professional development/skill updating Adequate resourcing Accountability Leadership
Royal Liverpool	Management appointment criteria Management training and continuing professional development Induction and staff training Culture

Recruitment and selection procedures

Good recruitment and selection procedures are important for the proper protection of patients, other healthcare workers and the public as they ensure that people are qualified to do the job and have the right skills for today's complex healthcare world. The risks of making inappropriate appointments are seen in poor performance in the role, with increased risk of error, and in risks from failure to meet statutory obligations. But raising standards will also have a positive effect, by ensuring healthcare attracts the most talented people.

So how can processes be enhanced, to address the lessons to be learnt from Allitt and others, and to ensure trusts appoint good people to all healthcare roles?

The purpose of recruitment is to attract applicants qualified for the jobs to be filled and the purpose of selection is to match applicants to those jobs. Most healthcare organisations have clear procedures for the recruitment and selection process, but it is worth summarising key good practice elements and commenting on some of the NHS and social policy trends that must also be taken into account.

Job description

Before any decision is made to advertise a job, the need and requirements of the role must be identified. Failure to do this adequately will result in inappropriate, costly appointments, leading to low productivity and high labour turnover. Developing a clear job description at this stage, in consultation with colleagues, sets out the role and its responsibilities, taking account of any changes required in the light of organisational design, costs, overlap of responsibilities and clinical risk. There must be constant review of job content and workload to make sure job descriptions are kept up to date and address responsibilities, including for managing risk areas.

Person specification

The person specification is derived from the job description and sets out the essential and desirable criteria required in the employee. In the NHS this increasingly takes a 'competency' approach. The term competencies is used to describe work-related attributes such as the qualifications, skills, knowledge, experience and values that a person draws on in order to do their job well.

An accurate person specification is essential in order to attract people with the right qualifications, skills and experience. As we will see, the person specification is the basis for the rest of the procedure – if it is wrong, the rest of the procedure will also fail.

Attracting applicants

Employers must think about their strategy to reach the target recruitment market, and how to sell the job in the person specification to people with the appropriate skills and qualifications. Most healthcare posts are advertised nationally in professional journals – it is a legal requirement for NHS consultant posts to be advertised in a minimum of two national journals – but there is increasing use of executive search and other external services (see below).

Equal opportunities

Employers also have to balance the need to match people to the person specification with national initiatives to encourage diversity. Employers who apply diversity policies recognise that a workforce that includes people from different social, cultural and educational backgrounds, age groups and the disabled can enrich the organisation. Inclusion policies enhance organisational performance in that poor targeting or indirect discrimination does not exclude people with high expertise.

Advertisements, job descriptions and person specifications must be free from any bias in terms of race, age and sex discrimination, and from requirements unjustifiably excluding people with disabilities.

The recent NHS equal opportunities agreement, which aims to make equality and diversity part of everything the service does, requires open competition unless jobs are needed for redeployment – for example, to meet employer obligations regarding suitable alternative employment for employees at risk of redundancy, or if an employee becomes disabled. These policies, which meet legal obligations and ensure scarce skills are retained, have to be reconciled with clinical risk safeguards in placing people in new roles, achieved by training and good line management.

Selection process

The recent *Code of Practice for Ministerial Appointments to Public Bodies*[8] issued by the Office of the Commissioner for Public Appointments, identifies principles on which appointments must be based. These are:

- merit

- independent scrutiny

- equal opportunities

- probity

- openness and transparency

- proportionality

Applying these principles to healthcare appointments at all levels, in an appropriate way for the level of seniority and responsibility, will improve the quality of appointments and provide a strong defence to any later challenges. Processes must aim to deliver appointments on merit, meaning on the basis of how an individual's ability, experience and qualities match up to the person specification, with an appropriate degree of objective assessment.

In practical terms this means objective shortlisting processes to determine who will be selected for interview. Applicants should be matched to the person specification criteria by means of a scoring system, and the outcome recorded.

Effective interviews

It also means that the selection process itself must be designed to identify the candidates who are qualified to do the job. There has been much criticism of the interview as a selection tool, because of the risk of failure to recognise deliberate inaccuracies in applications. Despite this, it remains the most common process in the NHS, mainly because there is still felt to be no substitute for face-to-face discussion with prospective employees.

The effectiveness of the interview can be improved by four factors:

- adequate training for panel members in equal opportunities and interview skills

- structured interviews based on the person specification – research shows that structured interviews – that is, those which follow a set pattern of questioning – have a higher success rate

- objective scoring systems, again based on the person specification

- including other appropriate selection tools – for example, presentations, group discussions, written, skill and psychometric tests

Any selection tools used in addition to the interview must be relevant to the job, justifiable, and fair in terms of equality legislation.

Following this process enhances objectivity and provides a robust mechanism for identifying the most suitable candidates. However, it will not in itself protect an organisation against the risk of an unsafe appointment. Processes must be used to establish the credentials of potential employees – as recommended by the reports on Allitt and others.

Credentialling

It has been estimated that as many as one in eight people exaggerate or falsify their qualifications or other information in their application. *Assuring the quality of medical practice*[9] states that in every sector of care it is a first principle to check, at the point of recruitment, that all professionals meet the high standards expected by the public. These checks are called 'credentialling', and they establish that the applicant is who they say they are, has the qualifications and references required, and does not have a record of poor performance which would call their suitability into question.

Checks

The checks are as follows:

- **Qualifications and professional registration** detailed in the application form should be checked with the registration or examination body before employment. Candidates should bring original certificates with them to interview to be checked by the recruitment specialist.

- **Any publications, prizes or awards** detailed in the application should be backed by evidence brought to interview.

- **Proof of identity,** preferably a passport, should be brought to interview. The photograph and information will verify proof of identity, but also serves to check the candidate has the right to live and work in the UK in accordance with the *Immigration and Asylum Act 1996.*

- **Satisfactory references** are needed from the present or most recent employer. Recruiters should validate the identity of referees, and whether they are representative of the person's career history and professional competence.

239

- **Criminal convictions** should be declared and suitability to work with children and vulnerable adults verified.

- **Fitness to practise** – for doctors, a health service circular[10] requires NHS employers to obtain a declaration covering any past or pending investigations by a regulatory body or the police. This must be confirmed at interview and any declarations discussed and considered before a decision on employment is made.

- **Pre-employment health assessment** – applicants should be cleared by occupational health departments.

Further guidance on references, criminal conviction and occupational health checks is given below.

Good practice for employers is to have a checklist of items for each candidate, and systems for picking up and dealing with problems. In the NHS this checklist must be kept up to date and incorporate any future national or statutory requirements. Particular note should be taken of the anticipated Data Protection Code of Practice, and of the impact of human rights rulings on employee rights to privacy and access to information in the pre-employment checking process.

Guidance on references

The purpose of references is to obtain information in confidence from a third party, providing a factual check on a candidate's employment history, qualifications, experience and suitability for the post. References are an essential part of the credentialling process, and must be viewed by appointment panels before a decision on employment is made.

Reliability

However, it would be misleading to assume that references are always reliable and provide all the information a prospective employer needs. References, like interviews, are one of the most frequently used predictors of candidate suitability, despite research showing validity and reliability problems. References in unstructured letter format can be subjective, telling us more about the referee than about the candidate. References can also be biased in terms of race or sex, and omit vital information about capability and fitness to practise.

Objectivity and accuracy

Employers today are more aware of the value of objective references from other employers, particularly in the same healthcare sector. However, they are also aware of recent cases that highlight the dangers of giving inaccurate or misleading references. Negligence claims can arise when facts provided in a reference are not properly checked, and an employer may be in breach of their duty of care to an employee if they fail to confine the reference to factually indisputable statements – for example, by referring to allegations which had not been substantiated.

However, there may also be a breach of the duty of care to other employers if a full and accurate reference is not given. Best guidance is to ensure that a reference, even if factually accurate, does not give an unfair impression of the former employee concerned.

Procedure

Developing a structured reference form, with forced choice options, and careful scrutiny of referee information can reduce these problems. If the panel does not view references until after the interview, objectivity can be improved. This reduces 'halo effect', particularly if panels also score candidates first. You can then see whether references support the ranking. The recruitment specialist should view the references before the interview in case there are issues to be followed up with referees or professional bodies, and of which the interviewers should be aware before they see the candidate.

To protect themselves from negligence or other claims, employers must provide guidance to senior managers on who can provide references and on the content.

Criminal convictions and protection of the public

Declaration of convictions

To safeguard the public, especially children and vulnerable adults, there are exemptions from the *Rehabilitation of Offenders Act 1974* enabling health employers to require applicants for jobs involving direct contact with patients to declare any convictions, whether spent or not under the Act. Employers have well-established procedures to check any declarations at the recruitment stage, and consider whether the nature or timing of the offence makes an applicant unsuitable for the job in question. To reduce the risk of inaccurate or undeclared offences, recruiters must check that declarations have been completed before shortlisting, and ask applicants to confirm they have no convictions at interview. They must also ask about any gaps in employment, and scrutinise references. If there are offences declared, these must be discussed at interview.

Further checks

More detailed checks must also be made on the possible criminal background of potential employees in regulated positions involving the care of children, young persons, or vulnerable adults. The Criminal Records Bureau has been set up to facilitate safer recruitment to protect these groups by making such information more accessible depending upon the nature of the work. The detail of the arrangements is yet to be finalised, but health organisations must now register with the bureau to obtain enhanced and standard disclosures to replace the current police checks.

In addition, under the *Protection of Children Act 1999*, childcare organisations must check names against the statutory lists when proposing to appoint someone to a childcare position, to ensure they are not disqualified from such work. Employers must refer names for possible inclusion if an employee harms a child, or puts them at risk of harm, in the course of employment.

Managers must note that they may be committing an offence under the *Criminal Justice and Court Services Act 2000* if they offer work, or allow someone to continue to work in a regulated position, in the knowledge that they are disqualified from such work. It is possible they may also be liable if there are adverse incidents arising from a failure to make appropriate checks.

Review

The *Rehabilitation of Offenders Act* is 25 years old, and under review as there are concerns about whether it strikes the right balance between fairness to ex-offenders and the need to protect the public. Meanwhile, the Criminal Records Bureau advises that recruiters must be fully aware of their duties under all relevant legislation. Ultimately it is the responsibility of the employer to decide whether to offer an applicant a job and it is worth remembering that criminal record checks and disclosures are no substitute for thorough pre-employment checks and good interview practice.

Pre-employment occupational health screening

Pre-employment occupational health screening is an essential risk management element of the recruitment and selection process. This is to facilitate:

- identification of people whose health background or personality profile may make them a danger to patients, the public or colleagues

- identification of existing ill-health which could be aggravated by work duties

- any adjustments to the duties and responsibilities, or terms and conditions required under the *Disability Discrimination Act 1995*

- identifying any employees needing follow up referrals

- ensuring new employees have the appropriate immunisation status

Good practice processes in pre-employment health screening include the following:

- A pre-employment health assessment carried out by the occupational health service (OHS) for all healthcare workers.

- Completion of a standard health questionnaire screened by the OHS, with an interview to assess fitness for the post if necessary.

- Details of the applicant's sickness record for the past year – this should be on the personal details/equal opportunities section of the application, seen only by the recruitment specialist to ensure confidentiality. This record should be verified with the previous employer, but note that care must be taken to ensure new data protection rules are not infringed.

- A question at interview to check any absence patterns or discrepancies, and that the applicant does not consider themselves disabled and require adjustments to be considered.

- Obtaining clearance from the occupational health department before an offer of employment is made.

Extreme cases

The Clothier report looked at the problem of picking up extreme cases through occupational health clearance because of the difficulty of assessing psychological health, in particular, personality disorder. The report concluded that excessive absence through sickness, excessive use of counselling or medical facilities, and self-harming behaviour such as attempted suicide, self-laceration and eating disorders are better guides than psychological testing.

From a common-sense point of view, any of these factors are likely to affect competence and performance in past jobs. Careful scrutiny of applications by trained recruiters should identify career or skill gaps and excessive sickness. Good probing questions at interview, covering the technical aspects of the role, past experience and competency scenarios may well exclude high-risk people on grounds of failure to meet the person specification.

Avoiding discrimination

In making decisions on grounds of excessive sickness absence or other health factors, selection panels must be careful not to discriminate against disabled applicants. Unreasonable failure to appoint on grounds of disability is unlawful under the *Disability Discrimination Act 1995*. All NHS employers must now have obtained the Employment Service's Two Ticks disability award, which means any disabled candidate who meets the person specification is offered an interview.

Duty of confidentiality

Occupational health departments must be provided with a copy of the job description and person specification both to assess adjustments needed in the case of a disability, but also to assess suitability for the job in general. Normally any discussions and outcomes remain confidential, and the manager is only told what is reasonable to be disclosed, but what does an occupational health specialist do if they find a real issue of concern? Should they break confidentiality to the individual, in order to protect patients, fellow professionals and the public generally?

The Bullock report examined the legal and professional code of ethics position in some detail, and concluded that there is no absolute duty of confidentiality. The public interest, as well as the interests of patients, can warrant, in appropriate and justifiable circumstances, disclosure of information. This principle is particularly important when managers refer employees for occupational health assessment because of sickness absence, performance concerns that may be health-related, or other problems arising in the course of employment.

Smart cards

An initiative that will help speed up health clearance on appointment, particularly in locum appointments, and with the transfer of reliable information between employers, is the NHS occupational health smart card pilot scheme. Smart cards will record pre-employment check data, including occupational health and immunisation records. This improvement in portability acknowledges that at present duplicate checks can be time-consuming for health workers who regularly move within the service – for example, for training – and also potentially costly for employers.

During the three-year pilot programme, doctors in training will be issued with personalised smart cards containing the doctor's name and photograph. All data will be securely stored but accessible to authorised personnel at any time. As the card will also record data on suitability to work in regulated positions and criminal record checks, recruiters will have immediate confirmation of a doctor's clearance for dealing safely with patients.

Other health issues

Employers are responsible for ensuring health workers, including locums and agency staff, have the correct immunisation status for the jobs they are to do. Healthcare workers who lack immunity must not perform exposure prone clinical procedures.

In this situation, variations in contracts of employment must be achieved by agreement with the individual, and if termination of employment is the only option, fair processes must be followed to avoid the risk of dismissal claims.

The report on the Elwood case (see p230) recommends particular attention to the occupational health assessment of older doctors. Care should be taken not to discriminate against older workers in any systems introduced. A better policy is to ensure clearance is obtained in the same way for all new employees, whether permanent or temporary, and that all employees and managers have access to good occupational health advice during employment.

External recruitment services

There are three main ways in which external recruitment services are used in healthcare:

- to provide specialist temporary workers on a regular basis (mainly nurses and locum doctors)

- to obtain short-term cover where internal solutions are not available (mainly administrative and clerical staff)

- for executive search in key or hard-to-fill senior posts (for example, chief executives or medical directors)

Staff shortages and an increasing preference from workers for the more flexible employment arrangements agency work can offer means agencies are playing an increasing role in shaping the healthcare workforce. Many employers have come to rely on external agencies to meet their staffing needs.

Agencies' obligations

The present law sets out minimum standards of conduct for employment agencies: agencies should check workers have the qualifications required by law for the job they are to do, and should obtain enough information to show a worker is suitable for the job. Higher standards to protect the public are proposed, including better checking of qualifications to ensure workers are not sent to do work which puts their and others' health and safety at risk because it is outside their experience or competence. Agencies will have to obtain references where temporary workers will be in regulated positions with children or vulnerable adults.

Many health employers already require this of agencies in service specifications. However, in practice experience shows reliance on this is not enough and employers must make their own checks. Incidents may not have been reported, and may only come to light through enquiries of previous employers. Good practice is to carry out pre-employment checks in the same way as you would for permanent staff.

Casual worker banks

Many acute trusts have tried to overcome this problem (and also cut costs in agency fees) by establishing their own casual worker banks, particularly for nurses, administrative and secretarial staff. This enables employers to check qualifications, registration and previous experience when people first join the bank, and to keep track of their capability. However bank staff, like agency workers, often do not have access to training and are not able to keep their skills up to date in the same way as permanent staff, and the casual nature of their employment means their contribution to the workforce is not maximised.

NHS Professionals

NHS Professionals, a programme that aims to combine the flexibility of agency and bank work with the benefits and perceived greater safety of NHS employment, is being rolled out across the NHS with the aim of resolving these issues.

Probationary contracts

Probationary periods of employment are often used in the health service where an occupational health review is required, but their main value is to enable an employer to assess whether a new employee is truly suitable for the job. This is especially valuable for clinical governance and assuring the quality of care, but there are pitfalls to be avoided in making appointments on a probationary basis.

Legal pitfalls

The pitfalls are partly legal – for example, failing to make it clear that employment is not guaranteed for the probationary period, but may be terminated by notice. If there is a need to terminate a contract before the end of the probationary period, then notice and operation of any disciplinary procedures must be in accordance with the contract. To avoid extending employment unnecessarily, notice periods while on probation should be shorter than for permanent employees, and there should be a shorter, less complex disciplinary procedure.

Managerial pitfalls

The other pitfalls are managerial: there is no point in having a probationary period if managers fail to monitor an employee's progress and to take action if it is not satisfactory, as once the probationary period expires it becomes a permanent contract. Probationary periods are generally three or six months, which is often not long enough to assess an individual, particularly in a complex role. They may also affect recruitment, as people in permanent jobs take a risk when accepting posts which are subject to satisfactory completion of a probationary period.

For all these reasons, probationary contracts are not widely used in NHS organisations, and employers rely on monitoring and action to improve performance, followed by normal capability or disciplinary procedures and appeal arrangements if the progress of a new employee is not satisfactory. Care must, however, be taken to initiate any action promptly, as delay in operating procedures may mean that employees have built up the one-year qualifying period for complaint to an employment tribunal. Procedures must always be operated fully and fairly, even if the employee has less than one year's service, as complaints may still be brought on grounds of sex, race, disability, pregnancy, maternity, trade union membership or certain aspects of industrial action, without the need for a qualifying period of employment.

Induction training programmes

There has been increasing recognition of the importance of induction courses and the initial settling-in period for employee retention, motivation and embedding safe working practices. Considerable time and effort is devoted to recruitment and selection processes, and an unsuccessful appointment, recent research by outplacement consultants Sanders and Sidney has found, can affect corporate momentum, as well as increase costs and personal distress.[11]

The employee is one of the variables in the risk management monitoring model. Induction is one way of raising employee awareness of how they can influence quality and make a real difference to the management of risk.

The way in which employees are received into an organisation is a crucial factor in forming their attitudes and ensuring they reach the required high standard of performance. This is the time when cultural issues, like the importance of teamworking and respect for patients raised in the Bristol inquiry, can be reinforced, and the risks associated with care provision reduced.

Corporate induction

Good practice is to have a corporate induction programme attended by all new employees within two months of starting work. A typical programme might include:

- introduction by the chief executive
- key issues for the organisation
- mission and standards
- human resource policies
- health and safety
- fire and emergency procedures

Key issues discussed can include human resource areas identified by risk management assessment, for example pre-employment checks or appraisal.

Local induction

In addition, managers must develop local induction programmes to meet the needs of new employees in the work area. The main benefits of this approach are:

- New employees settle in quickly and become productive early.
- Motivation is increased and maintained.
- Employee turnover, lateness, absenteeism and poor performance may be reduced.
- It helps to develop a management style where the emphasis is on leadership.
- Employees work in a safer environment.

Time with line managers

It is important that new employees meet and spend time with their colleagues in the first days and understand the culture. Research suggests that, when employees leave a job early, most cited getting on with the boss as a crucial factor. It is important to arrange quality time with the line manager, when standards and responsibility can be reinforced, as this is where most problems are likely to occur.

Disaffected people are probably also those who may give rise to risk – for example, from failure to follow procedures fully or to the best of their ability.

Organisations must have a checklist of items for managers to go through during the first day. Typically these include: terms and conditions of employment, duties and responsibilities, standards and rules of conduct, health and safety, and confidentiality. In a busy department, with staff shortages, it is easy to skimp on local, initial induction. This is poor practice, providing another example of how short cuts can open up risk for the organisation.

The NHS places particular importance on induction for newly qualified medical and dental staff and for doctors joining another hospital or moving to another speciality. Induction courses are compulsory for pre-registration posts and must cover management issues, professional concerns such as death certification, breaking bad news, and keeping GPs informed of their patients' progress.

Addressing poor clinical performance

The NHS consultation document *Supporting doctors, protecting patients*[12] on preventing, recognising and dealing with poor clinical performance of doctors was published in response to a number of recent inquiries, particularly Bristol, and public concern. Acknowledging the need for change, the document also pictures success, stating that over the past decade the demands on doctors have changed substantially. These include workload pressures, higher public and patient expectations, advances in technology, new responsibilities to meet explicit clinical standards and greater emphasis on training. The document states: "Doctors have shown remarkable ability to rise to these challenges and, year after year, the majority deliver a first-class service to their patients."

Key lessons

The growing number of cases of poor clinical performance hitting the headlines has important lessons for skill updating, which are just as applicable to non-clinical staff. Key lessons include:

- Although many cases were presented as a single incident, when investigated it was clear that a pattern of poor practice had developed over a long period of time.

- Although such problems may not have been officially recognised, they were often known about in informal networks.

- Systems that might have been expected to detect poor outcomes of care and weak processes had failed to pick up problems with the practice of the doctor concerned.

The document cites in particular the Bristol inquiry and the further case of a gynaecologist dismissed by South Kent Hospitals NHS Trust in early 1996 because of apparent serious failures in clinical practice.

Unsatisfactory disciplinary procedures

The human resource function has a key role where suspension and dismissal is concerned, but the *Revitalising* consultation document found important failings in the operation of disciplinary procedures. Few medical disciplinary procedures emphasise the need to involve the human resources function at an early stage for professional employment advice. As a result, procedures do not provide proper protection for patients, are cumbersome and costly to operate, and are not always fair to doctors. The report says: "Over-reliance is placed on disciplinary solutions to problems late in the day, whilst mechanisms to produce earlier remedial and educational solutions are particularly weak."

So what are the remedial and educational solutions recommended and currently being put in place by health employers?

Continuing professional development (CPD)

CPD programmes are the means by which healthcare professionals and managers ensure their knowledge and skills are up to date. As an example, in future all consultants will have to show evidence of personal development plans and action on CPD as part of the appraisal process operated by employers and for revalidation by the General Medical Council (GMC).

Human resource practitioners have a key role in the introduction of CPD for doctors in their organisation, and in the employment issues when remedial training or other action is needed. While remedial training is ongoing, human resource practitioners will have to resolve alternative employment, job plan revisions and adjustments to contracts of employment, in consultation with clinical directors, individual doctors and their staff representative.

Appraisal

Appraisal has been a feature of managing senior and administrative health workers for some time, but as several of the reports found, is less embedded for clinicians.

The NHS Plan announced the intention that all doctors employed or under contract to the NHS will, as a condition of contract, be required to participate in annual appraisal from 2001. Appraisal is defined in *Supporting doctors, protecting patients* as a positive process to give feedback on performance, chart continuing progress and identify development needs. It is a forward-looking process essential for the developmental and educational planning needs of an individual.

Individual responsibility for risk

However, to address risk, the appraisal and personal development plan process must include an assessment of individual responsibility for risk. This should be based on quantitative and qualitative data on performance, and identify the lessons learned from errors or untoward outcomes.

As an example, the consultant appraisal scheme is described as a professional process of constructive dialogue, in which the doctor being appraised has a formal structured opportunity to reflect on their work and consider how their performance might be improved. The scheme content focuses on clinical aspects of the consultant's work, including audit activity reports, any investigations following complaints, risk management, professional relationships with patients and colleagues, and teamworking.

The problem for the human resource professional and the manager is to make sure all this happens; that comprehensive annual appraisals do take place and that outcomes are realistic and pursued.

To this extent, the problems of appraisal for consultants are no different to those for other health workers; there is an equal need for appraisal in the case of nurses (as shown by the Clothier and Bullock reports) and other health professionals and managers, as there is for the most junior administrative and clerical staff. Good appraisal will have an impact on quality of care and reduction of risk.

Revalidation

Assuring the quality of medical practice[9] considers the contribution of self-regulation as exercised by the GMC. The current system determines who should enter and remain in the profession at different levels and in different fields of practice, helping organisations achieve high quality standards through clinical governance.

Following concerns about the ability of the GMC to act swiftly and effectively when a doctor's fitness to practise is called into question and risk arises, new legislation has been introduced which provides for interim suspension orders to stop a doctor practising, and imposes a duty on the GMC to notify employers and others of doctors whose fitness to practise is under consideration. There is also now a five-year period before a doctor who has been struck off the GMC's medical register can apply for re-registration.

The GMC is introducing a revalidation process that will require all doctors to demonstrate on a regular basis that they continue to be fit to practise. Revalidation will be linked to NHS appraisal schemes, but requires legislation to make participation mandatory.

Referrals

Supporting doctors, protecting patients confirms that employers have a public duty, beyond the employer-employee relationship, to report serious problems to the GMC independently of any disciplinary or other action taken by the employer. This is particularly important if the doctor is dismissed and is likely to practise elsewhere, as the GMC is the only body which can suspend or remove a doctor's registration and stop this happening. Referrals should also be made where there is evidence of false claims regarding qualifications, experience or publications.

Again, the position here is no different to other health professionals. The issue for human resource specialists is to ensure proper, prompt procedures for determining whether a referral should be made. Referral should only be made where an initial prompt investigation provides accurate, documented evidence of a case to answer. Special care must be taken to ensure there is no discrimination on grounds of race, sex, disability, or other unlawful grounds, and that confidentiality is observed.

Retraining in the light of lessons from incidents

Understanding how risk arises, and the consequences of working where risk may arise, is a learning process. Organisations must understand the causes of risk, and its link with quality.

Learning from people management failures, adverse incidents and near-misses in organisations is very important for organisational development and business success. John Peters, the Gulf War veteran, says in an article in the journal *People Management*:

"Individual trial and error is a very ineffective way to learn. It is infinitely better to learn from someone else's mistakes rather than your own. If companies can create an open culture where people feel safe admitting their mistakes, then corporate wisdom will grow dramatically."[13]

There is enormous potential for development here, supported by the Health and Safety Executive (HSE), which has found an unacceptably high number of employers do not have proper procedures in place for assessing the causes of accidents and learning from them.[14] In the NHS, there is to be a single national system of reporting adverse patient events and near-misses through the National Patient Safety Agency.

OWAM recommendations

The NHS report *An Organisation with a Memory* (see KEY REFERENCES, piii) addresses the need for a national system to identify and learn effectively from incidents. It advocates a change in culture towards reporting by encouraging more open and blame-free approaches, to ensure that lessons learnt in one part of the organisation are properly shared with the whole.

The main human resources recommendations from this report are the need for:

• a more open culture, in which errors or service failures can be reported and discussed

• mechanisms for ensuring that, where lessons are identified, the necessary changes are put into practice

Learning from incidents and complaints needs to be an integral feature of appraisal systems, with individual retraining needs identified and incorporated in personal development plans. Where learning from incidents indicates a wider organisational need, the required changes must be incorporated in induction programmes, education and training courses. This is particularly relevant to cultural issues. Other lessons are the need for more effective training management, teambuilding and leadership.

Leadership and management development

All healthcare organisations should have leadership development plans in place and resources identified to provide support for leaders at all levels. The NHS human resources framework states that this must focus on personal leadership qualities, effective organisational and system leadership, thus improving clinical quality, and leading modernisation programmes. Nationally, this is being rolled out through the NHS Leadership Centre programme.

Understanding risk

Part of improving clinical quality is reducing the adverse effect of risk. Leadership is important for risk management, in terms of ensuring a well-run organisation with high care standards, but also to introduce and develop risk management as a concept into the organisation and to provide a constant reminder of its value and of the consequences of not taking account of risk.

Similarly, management training programmes, which include decision-making, must consider the consequences of individual judgments and the impact on risk. In human resource terms, poor judgment often arises when established systems or routines are ignored or manipulated, often for short-term gain. Management development programmes must therefore include consideration of the rationale for a systems approach to high-risk areas, and an understanding of the flexibilities available, as well as the processes for introducing change. They must also include educating managers to be able to identify, assess and control risks.

An example of the effect of failure to do this lies in the area of harassment, particularly racial. If a manager fails to investigate whether this is an issue – by, for example, asking questions at appraisal – or fails to act on receipt of a complaint, disaffected people with reduced motivation may lay the organisation open to risk, or leave and complain to a tribunal. Yet this is an area where risks can be managed by effective harassment and diversity policies.

Senior management development

All healthcare organisations should also have management training strategies, which take on board the lessons from adverse incidents. Human resource professionals can have a key role in brokering senior management/board level development by:

- advising on development opportunities

- facilitating the arrangements – for example, by study leave policies or cover for the job

Useful approaches to senior management development include:

- outside organisation options – secondments, development programmes, academic courses

- mentoring, coaching and shadowing

- learning groups

- 360 degree feedback (from colleagues, subordinates and managers)

- e-learning

Creating a learning organisation, where training needs at all levels, including senior managers and professionals, are addressed, is essential for benefiting from mistakes or near-misses and poor practice.

High-performance, patient-centred teams

There is increasing recognition that high-quality patient-centred care relies upon effective teamworking across traditional skill groups and staff boundaries.

Why teams fail

Teams fail where there is:

- a lack of mutual respect, trust and openness

- little understanding of individual differences

- a source of unresolved conflict

Teambuilding exercises with an external facilitator can help address these problems.

Team bonus pilots

In the NHS, team bonus pilots are being introduced to identify the most effective ways of rewarding and incentivising high-quality performance. The pilots aim to test how far team based rewards help to:

- clarify goals and priorities at team and organisational level
- encourage cooperative work and behaviour

The premise is that individual bonuses can be divisive, while team bonuses can strengthen links between colleagues and encourage more collaborative work.

Importance of adequate resources

In managing risk, it has to be accepted that additional resources may be needed. One of the present main areas of concern is the effect of staffing shortages on maintenance and development of services.

Staff shortages

The report on the Bristol inquiry says that the inquiry team was "sometimes amazed" that the paediatric cardiac service could be maintained at all, such was the staff shortage. Specialist cardiologists and surgeons were found to be below a proper level and lacked junior support. According to the report, understaffing was so great that the cardiologists could not participate effectively in surgery or intensive care. There was a shortage of nurses trained in care of children, theatre work and intensive care.

The NHS Plan recognises that one of the biggest constraints facing the delivery of healthcare today is human resources. The only way the modernisation agenda and patient-centred care will be delivered is by greater investment in frontline staff. The Plan proposes increases in the number of consultants, GPs and nurses, but it will take several years before resource investment pays off.

Initiatives to increase numbers

There are a number of initiatives in hand to increase numbers in the short term. One is the national advertising campaign to encourage trained nurses and other healthcare professionals who have left to return. Return-to-practice refresher courses and assigned mentors have been successful in returning many former employees. Flexible working arrangements and nursery provision under the Improving Working Lives Standard[15] encourages this.

Under the NHS Professionals programme, nurses can work shift patterns that suit them and are supported by training and skill updating. Self-rostering arrangements have had considerable success in boosting staff availability for work and contributing to adequate resourcing.

International recruitment

International recruitment is another major central strategy. Several recent surveys have pointed to a general skill shortage in the UK, and many organisations are looking to import staff. Looking globally makes business sense, but raises ethical issues about the impact on home and developing country labour markets and economies. The NHS Executive agreed in 1999 that it would not recruit from countries that were themselves facing shortages of health professionals, especially poorer nations. International nurse recruitment has therefore been targeted at countries where there is a recognised surplus of health staff.

There are risks involved. Nurses arriving in the UK attend cultural adaptation courses to improve their English and their knowledge of UK health systems of care, and provide advice on issues such as setting up bank accounts and finding accommodation. Expert teams trained in credentialling professionals from other countries are needed to recruit them. Further risks are associated with recruiting individuals from countries with endemic infectious disease, particularly in relation to involvement in exposure-prone procedures.

The Government is now looking to recruit consultants and GPs from countries such as Spain that have a doctor surplus.[16] A recent British Medical Association press statement supporting the initiative advised on ways to reduce clinical governance risks. This said: "It is imperative that doctors coming to work in the UK are offered structured induction programmes and support to enable them to settle into practice."

Balanced skill mix

Having the right skill mix in the workforce is important in healthcare. This is primarily for cost reasons – healthcare is labour intensive and its people account for a high proportion of total costs. Second, it is important for quality improvement, which in turn reduces the risk of errors. In a time of skill shortage, changes to skill mix, and the development of a more flexibly skilled workforce is crucial for achieving improvements in clinical practice.

What is meant by skill mix? A recent discussion paper for the World Health Organisation[17] describes the variations in definition. The term can refer to the mix of posts in the establishment, the mix of employees in a post, the combination of skills available at a specific time, or, alternatively, it may refer to the combination of activities in each role.

For the NHS, interest in skill mix is prompted by the need to fill the gap caused by a shortage in supply of staff. The approach to skill mix review is therefore to explore alternative staffing solutions, such as redesigning roles or skill substitution. It is also prompted by new approaches to care organisations, such as patient-focused care, and partnership working with social services departments, the independent and voluntary sectors.

Alternative staffing solutions

Expanding the role of nurses to use their skills and experience in tasks traditionally carried out by doctors was set out as a key objective in the NHS Plan. Specialist nurses in NHS trusts now book patients into their own operating lists and carry out minor operations. In orthopaedics, for example, this can reduce waiting times for patients with minor conditions.

Specialist GPs are also starting to carry out minor surgery and diagnostic procedures to speed up waiting times for their patients and release pressure on local hospitals. They can filter out cases they can deal with, and make sure a consultant sees urgent or complicated cases.

The need for greater consultant-led services – for example, 24-hour cover in labour wards – means redesigning services and the mix of staff and roles in the teams providing the service. Teams in obstetrics can include a mix of specialist consultants, staff grade doctors, senior house officers or specialist registrars, and nurse or midwife practitioners. This offers better training for doctors and continuity of expert care for patients.

NHS Direct

NHS Direct is a further example of achieving better skill mix and safer care by freeing up frontline staff. Routing telephone calls to accident and emergency departments to NHS Direct mean nurses can now spend more time with patients.

Staff retention

Staff retention is another essential feature of adequate resourcing for the modernisation programme and safe systems of care. Many qualified staff leave to work abroad, or for family reasons. Failing to keep staff can be costly in terms of replacement, but the organisation also loses valuable skills, knowledge and experience, often gained by years of expensive training. In some medical specialties this is currently irreplaceable.

There is particular concern about attrition in training. The NHS performance framework gives targets to reduce attrition rates to 13% in pre-registration nursing and midwifery training, and 10% in pre-registration therapist training.

Boosting retention

So how can an employer boost retention? Good induction, as shown earlier (see pp248–250), is invaluable. Paying the going rate is also important – financial packages must be fair and motivating, based on pay market data and job evaluation. Good human resource policies provide a framework for employees to work within and understand what is expected of them. Essential core policies are discipline and grievance, health and safety, trade union recognition and consultation. However, development and training opportunities, and recognition, are just as important for retention, and human resource strategy must include personal development plans for each employee, balancing the needs of the organisation with a rewarding role and meeting employment expectations.

Flexible working

The NHS Improving Working Lives Standard[15] recognises the value of a well-managed, flexible working environment that supports staff, promotes their welfare and development and provides a productive work-life balance. In a predominantly female workforce, having a range of family-friendly policies can also boost retention. The good healthcare employer will have in place policies on flexible working, such as part-time working, jobsharing and homeworking, special and carer leave, maternity, paternity and parental leave, nursery and out-of-school care places.

Morale

Media headlines are full of references to low morale in organisations and its impact on safety. In healthcare, low morale is attributed in media reports to many factors including high stress levels, racism, poor staffing levels and working conditions. Low morale is one of the reasons why people leave their jobs. Investing in staff can boost productivity by increasing morale and lowering staff turnover, and can also improve patient satisfaction.

Measuring and improving morale

Morale can be defined as the confidence, enthusiasm and discipline of a person or group at a particular time. So how can morale be properly gauged, and what sort of staff investment will make a difference? Use of annual staff attitude surveys enables employers to identify the things employees think they do well, and those which require improvement. This tool can help measure progress in improving the quality of working life for staff. Further action in the areas identified can in turn improve retention, motivation and quality of care.

Two areas employers are increasingly looking to invest in, with the aim of directly impacting on morale and motivation, are communications and staff involvement.

Employee communication

Employee communication is well recognised as an important action area in times of restructuring, mergers or cost reduction. Organisational morale can be particularly low when people are waiting to hear how jobs will be filled in the new organisation, who will be transferred and which jobs may no longer be required. As well as maintaining work levels during times of turbulence, employers are anxious to retain skills during the transition. In the case of most healthcare roles, these are key skill areas that will be needed in the new organisation.

Communication strategies are also important for projecting key messages about risk management and good practice in patient care. All health organisations should have an employee communications strategy setting out how people will be kept up to date with key developments and able to input their own views and questions. Communication mechanisms, some of which may seem fairly obvious, include:

- face-to-face dialogue – small or large groups, and an open door policy

- mechanisms for structured feedback from employees and evidence that this is listened to, for example, working and focus groups, question and answer sheets

- briefings – organisational and team, by e-mail, notice boards and other communication systems

- training and awareness raising

- websites

- distribution of letters, memos, meeting notes, annual reports

- newsletters, bulletins, news sheets

- telephone hotlines, confidential counselling service

These methods need to be evaluated to decide which types are most effective for the message to be conveyed.

Staff involvement

Good communication up, down and across the organisation is one of the key outcomes of a staff involvement strategy. An involving, open culture, where everyone understands the organisation's goals, is an important part of fostering a sense of belonging and raising standards. Staff involvement, including partnership working with trade unions, networks and working groups, to enable staff to participate in care practice development, and organisational development are also important.

Sickness absence

High sickness absence in an organisation is another factor hindering strategies for adequate resourcing. Absence rates vary between different types of health professionals, but sickness absence has the same effect of depriving teams of key skills which often have to be covered at short notice by locum, bank or agency staff.

A survey by the Chartered Institute of Personnel and Development (CIPD)[18] has put the cost of sickness absence at £487 per employee per year, or £12 billion to the economy as a whole. UK workers take an average 8.7 days sickness absence per year, but the majority of employers surveyed believed that around one-third of this was not due to actual ill-health. Many employers also believed there was significant under reporting of time off.

Effective sickness absence policies

It goes without saying therefore that health employers can make considerable cost savings, and improve the quality of healthcare, by effective sickness absence policies. Effective management of the health and welfare of people at work can contribute to performance improvement as well as lowering absenteeism, improving morale and reducing litigation costs associated with ill-health and industrial injuries. Family-friendly and flexible working policies are also important for providing the means for people to manage childcare and other domestic crises without 'going sick'.

The features of an effective sickness absence policy include:

- monitoring of absence by managers, with triggers for investigation
- return to work interviews with managers to identify poor attendance and occupational causes
- mechanisms for referral to occupational health services
- fair processes for dealing with persistent short-term absence
- procedures for handling alternative employment, rehabilitation and, if necessary, capability dismissals due to long-term ill-health

Rehabiliation and disability

All aspects of the procedure must comply with the provisions of the *Disability Discrimination Act 1995*. Where action is being taken concerning employees whose illness or condition brings them within the scope of the Act, the employer will have to show that it has not discriminated against the employee as a result of their disability. It is essential in cases of long-term ill-health to offer any alternative employment that the employee can do, making reasonable adjustments in accordance with the Act, and case managing rehabilitation into work.

Stress at work

Stress is one of the most frequent causes of sickness absence at work, aggravated in healthcare by staff shortages, violence against staff and the demands of the roles. Occupational stress poses a risk to all businesses, illustrated by a number of high profile cases of claims for damages caused by work-related stress. The HSE considers occupational stress to be the second most common work-related illness after back pain, estimated to be responsible for 6.5 million lost working days in the UK each year.

As discussed in chapter 6, employers have a general duty under health and safety legislation to undertake risk assessments and manage activities to reduce the risk to employees from stress in their jobs. To avoid the risks of claims, and reduce the risks to the organisation from behaviour associated with stress, health employers must have stress management policies in place. These should help identify the causes of stress, aim to minimise them and provide employees with a counselling service for confidential advice and support.

Counselling

Health organisations are increasingly realising the value of employee assistance, or counselling services in a number of high-risk situations. In an environment where jobs are stressful, confidential, independent helpline services can support employees and provide them with access to the specialist advice they need to enable them to carry on with their roles. Part of this process will be helping employees to understand the risks to their own and others' safety, the possible consequences of those risks and how they can be minimised. Human resource policies aimed at avoiding violence at work for frontline staff – for example, ambulance and accident and emergency workers – addresses this.

Personal problems

Counselling, or employee assistance programmes, can also help people cope with personal problems, which may be affecting them at work as well as at home, and contribute to risk. These problems may include alcohol or drug abuse, relationship difficulties, ageing parents or financial worries. All employers should have human resource policies that enable them to deal sympathetically with employees with drug and alcohol problems, including referral to occupational health services, but that also manage the risk to patients and fellow workers.

Dealing with distress

Health organisations, particularly the emergency services, are in the frontline in major accidents and disaster scenarios. While teams of professionals are trained to deal with distressing situations, many emergency workers will still need access to counselling services to cope with their reactions. Employers who provide these are more likely to retain key staff, enable them to continue effectively in their specialist roles, and to manage the risks they face, or must make decisions about, every day.

People management of non-clinical staff

NHS national guidance reinforces the need for better human resource policies and strategy to support clinical governance and performance improvement. *Assuring the quality of medical practice* states:

> "We have always recognised that offering fast, quality care to patients and delivering modern and dependable services with courtesy and understanding means attracting and retaining high quality staff, committed to developing their skills and keeping them up to date."

This maxim applies as much to non-clinical health workers as to clinicians. Although most of the examples given so far in this chapter concern medical or nursing staff, it is worth remembering that a large proportion of health workers are non-clinical, including ancillary, scientific and technical, ambulance, administrative and clerical staff and senior managers. Many of the good practice processes described apply equally to them, as there are many non-clinical workers with access to patients or equipment, where risks may arise.

ODPs

Action to raise standards and manage risk is seen in the example of operating department practitioners (ODPs – formerly known as theatre technicians). Their professional association holds and maintains a register of operating department practitioners, with the aims of protecting the public and ensuring that all registered ODPs conform to a code of professional conduct and are fit to practise. There is a formal structure for dealing with complaints about conduct, and all health employers must now check with the register before employing ODPs.

Recruitment and selection

For all employees, it is important to carry out pre-employment checks, thorough induction, training and appraisal, and to learn from errors and risks. Although for many jobs there will not be a direct impact on patient care, there will almost certainly be an indirect effect. This can be seen, potentially, in failures to order equipment, to manage finances, or to route emergency calls correctly, for example.

Managers carry out most NHS recruitment and selection, although professionals are often involved in the process. Many managers in this role do not realise that they may have a personal liability for any adverse incidents resulting from failure to carry out pre-employment checks correctly, as well as the potential to involve their employer in risk and damage to public confidence. This is seen in the criticism of recruiters in several of the major reports.

The impact of under-investment in people

Healthcare organisations are highly complex, and weak links can have significant impact on frontline services – the effect, often, of shortcuts or under-investment in areas where a real difference can be made. An example of this is the current drive to improve ward cleanliness, a subject of frequent public criticism and a perceived measure of healthcare standards. Under-investment in the management and delivery of cleaning services is now being addressed, and seen as a key performance indicator for NHS trusts. Yet poor performance of individuals, high sickness absence and labour turnover can just as easily jeopardise this initiative and affect delivery of clinical services.

Similarly, in several pilot schemes, clerical and administrative workers are at the forefront of new hospital booking systems allowing patients to choose a date for their first appointment. Admissions booked in this way maximises slots available and can shorten waiting lists because patients are more likely to keep an appointment which suits them. This can have a positive impact on the productivity of frontline staff, but again can be jeopardised just as easily by poor people management.

New roles and policies

Family-friendly policies, training, particularly in information technology and computing, and good recruitment practice can equally enhance the efficiency and motivation of clerical staff in these kinds of roles. New roles are being created to reinforce this process of increasing people's contribution in the workplace. Childcare coordinators have a direct impact on sickness absence by helping staff find high quality, reliable childcare.

The NHS human resource performance framework introduces performance measures for employers to achieve in these areas, reiterating that the demonstration of how standards are met is increasingly seen as the way forward.

Discrimination and other claims

The statutory framework relevant to risk management is not confined to health and safety but includes other areas of employment law.

This chapter includes several references to risks arising from a failure to prevent unlawful discrimination on grounds of sex, race, and disability and gender reassignment, which current UK legislation specifically covers. Discrimination is a developing area of law, and employers must keep up to date, particularly with regard to discrimination on grounds of religion, age and sexual orientation, which are covered by the European framework directive. Cases have also been brought in these areas under the indirect discrimination provisions of current law.

Sex and race

Under the *Sex Discrimination Act 1975* and the *Race Relations Act 1976*, both direct and indirect discrimination in employment is unlawful.

Direct discrimination

As a broad summary, direct discrimination occurs when someone is treated unfavourably on grounds of sex, marital status or race in areas such as recruitment, training and promotion. Discrimination on racial grounds includes colour, race, and nationality, or ethnic or national origins. The *Race Relations Amendment Act 2000* places an additional duty on public authorities not to discriminate in carrying out their functions.

Indirect discrimination

Indirect discrimination is broadly where an employer imposes a requirement or condition in which

- the proportion of the relevant group that can comply is considerably smaller

- the employer cannot justify
- operates to the detriment of the individual concerned

The new *Sex Discrimination (Indirect Discrimination and Burden of Proof) Regulations 2001* replace "requirement or condition" in the case of indirect sex discrimination with "provision, criterion and practice". This more flexible wording means employers must review their employment practices, particularly in recruitment and promotion, to ensure people are treated fairly.

Legal challenges on indirect discrimination grounds have been successfully brought in a wide variety of cases, including shift changes, essential and desirable criteria in job advertisements, refusal to consider requests to work from home or part time, dress codes and age bars.

Disability

The *Disability Discrimination Act 1995 (DDA)* makes it unlawful for employers to treat a disabled person less favourably on the grounds of disability, without a justifiable reason. The *DDA* covers recruitment, selection and promotion, and recently has also been held to include selection for redundancy. Capability dismissal on grounds of ill-health will also probably be caught by the *DDA*, and fair procedures, including offers of alternative employment, must be followed.

To come under the protection of the *DDA*, a person must have a disability. This is defined as a physical or mental impairment, causing substantial and long-term effect on ability to carry out day-to-day activities. These definitions are being increasingly clarified by case law, and employers must ensure their corporate knowledge is kept up to date.

All employers must have policies to ensure risk reduction from unlawful discrimination acts by managers and staff. All managers must be trained in equality issues, ensure their actions do not infringe legislation and refer any issues arising for specialist human resource advice.

Harassment

An increasing area of challenge, which can affect morale and employee attraction and retention, is harassment on sexual or racial grounds. Unless employers have effective policies covering this, and act swiftly to deal with all instances of harassment, they are open to complaints of sex or race discrimination. Recent cases show costs can be high, particularly where there is in addition an award for injury to feelings arising out of unlawful discrimination, or a claim for compensation for psychiatric injury or stress.

Human rights

Employers must also take account of new legislation on civil liberties. The *Human Rights Act 1998* gives the right to challenge public authorities where they act in conflict with human rights. Employment-related rights protected include the right to freedom of expression, association and assembly, and to privacy and family life.

Power to investigate

The *Regulation of Investigatory Powers Act 2000* limits employers' rights to intercept employee e-mails, faxes and telephone calls, unless consent has been given or there is a legitimate business interest. Since increasing reliance is placed on e-mail as a prime means of business communication, this is a growing area of risk, but the new rules mean employers cannot rely on the right to take action on e-mail or internet abuse unless policy has been effectively communicated.

Whistleblowing

Under the *Public Interest Disclosure Act 1998*, an employee who blows the whistle on an employer's fraudulent or criminal activities has protection against victimisation, provided they follow prescribed routes. This will include protection for health workers in situations such as the Bristol case, and be important in the future for enabling unsafe processes to be identified and action taken before they become major issues. All NHS employers must have whistleblowing policies.

Excessive working hours

A key area of risk in clinical practice is long working hours. The *Working Time Regulations* came into force on 1 October 1998, implementing the European *Working Time Directive*. It is important to note that the Directive was adopted as a health and safety measure, to ensure minimum rest periods, leave entitlements and maximum weekly working hours protection for all workers.

Working Time Regulations

Under the Regulations, working time is limited to:

- an average of 48 hours a week over the reference period (generally 26 weeks)
- an average of eight hours in 24 for nightworkers

There are also the following rights:

- for nightworkers to receive free health assessments
- to 11 hours' rest in each 24 hours
- to a rest period of 24 hours in every seven days (or 48 hours in each 14 days)
- to an in-work rest break if the working day is longer than six hours
- to four weeks' paid leave per year from day one of employment

Impact on health organisations

These rights and obligations have had a considerable impact on the organisation of working time in health organisations, where groups of health workers have a variety of contractual arrangements, including shift and nightwork, on-call and standby, temporary and additional bank work, and overtime. Employers have had to adjust shift patterns and invest in additional employees, to ensure they are able to cover the service and provide the entitled breaks. This is a good example of where the needs of the service will not protect employers from possible prosecution if rest breaks are not provided; the only options are service reductions, with their own risks, or investment in staff.

Exceptions to the Regulations

It is the nature of healthcare provision that there will be instances where people will be needed to work beyond the limits – for example, consultants in operating theatres, radiographers called out at night and ambulance paramedics attending an emergency at the end of their shift. The Regulations allow for this in several ways, but there are risks for the employer in ensuring safe working practices.

By virtue of regulation 4, individual workers can, by written agreement, choose to disapply the weekly working hours limit. In addition, workers whose working time (or part of it) is not measured or predetermined are exempt from some provisions. However, the basis of the Regulations is that long hours are harmful to health. A failure to monitor working time, or to protect against excessive working, could therefore be used as evidence of a failure to provide a safe system of work if an employee brings a claim against their employer. *Johnstone and Bloomsbury Health Authority* (Court of Appeal 1991) illustrates this (see box).

In the health economy today, many doctors and other professionals still work exceptionally long hours to meet clinical need. Employers must ensure hours and health are monitored to avoid the risk of similar cases.

A case of excessive working hours

Dr Johnstone was a senior house officer employed under a contract of employment with a standard working week of 40 hours and, in addition, availability on call for a further 48 hours a week. He claimed that the authority was under a duty to take all reasonable care for his safety and well-being, and that they were in breach of that duty by requiring him to work intolerable hours. The Court of Appeal ruled that the authority could not lawfully require a doctor to work so much overtime in any week, as it was reasonably foreseeable that it would damage his health.

Rest periods

The Regulations also provide for derogation on rest periods in certain specified circumstances or where there is a collective agreement, provided that compensatory rest is given. In the case of career grade doctors, a derogation of some Regulations relating to nightworking and rest has been applied, subject to the provision of compensatory rest. Government guidance defines compensatory rest as a period of rest, the same length as the period of rest, or part of a period of rest, that a worker has missed.

The problem for health employers is ensuring that where there is entitlement to compensatory rest that this is given within a reasonable space of time, whilst protecting clinical activity such as theatre lists. NHS employers are developing local agreements on this in accordance with national guidance. However, it is clear that there is an expectation from the HSE, and healthcare professionals themselves, that these policies will ensure protection for workers and patients.

There are also problems for employers in preventing excessive hours working by employees with second jobs with another employer. This situation requires careful monitoring to protect patient care. If there is an effect on performance, then action should be taken under fair procedures.

Exit interviews

An exit interview is a conversation between a departing employee who is leaving either voluntarily or involuntarily, and a representative from the organisation. Although of benefit to employees as a means of identifying complaints, the real value of the exit interview is as a reality check for the employer, to see how the organisation is doing. In terms of risk management, the exit interview is a significant learning tool, with the opportunity to identify poor or unsafe practice, and to take action before public whistleblowing occurs.

The employee's line manager or supervisor should not conduct the exit interview, as they will almost certainly not be sufficiently objective, and may inhibit honest replies. In most cases, properly trained human resources staff are best suited for this role. Questions must be open ended, sensitive, neutral and tailored to each individual in order to identify particular concerns or inconsistencies.

What should the interview cover?

All exit interviews should be structured to check leaving arrangements, terms and conditions and attitudes to the organisation as an employer. However, an interview focusing on risk management must in particular cover:

- reasons for the termination or departure

- the supervisor's management skills

- any concerns about working practices

- how effectively the department operates

- any questionable practices connected with the termination or departure – for example, improper payments

Protecting the organisation

The exit interview also gives the organisation two further opportunities connected with risk management. One is to ensure the employee understands any continuing obligations about confidentiality, and returns any keys, security or identity cards, codes or healthcare property. There may also be a need to resolve any outstanding disputes, and explain policy on the provision of references. There may also be a need to protect the organisation by assessing whether the employee is high risk for any grudge action – for example, computer sabotage – or whether an alert warning to other employers is needed.

Staff retention issues

The second opportunity is to identify staff retention issues, particularly in areas of recruitment shortages, and how these may be addressed. The exit interview is the last opportunity to persuade people to stay, either in the same role or by redeployment in another area, or to return at a later date. Career break schemes, parental leave, elder care, study leave and secondments are all important elements in the make up of a good employer, and will be positive and much cheaper alternatives to offer to avoid the resignation of a valued employee.

Good practice in people management

The people issues of risk management in healthcare are constantly evolving, either because of legislative or case law developments, or as a result of changing government or NHS policy. It is essential that health employers keep up to date with these developments, and incorporate them in their policies and the day-to-day management of the organisation. Employers and managers must ensure they have all the relevant documentation, and seek expert human resources or legal advice, before taking action.

Key actions

So what, in summary are the key actions an employer can take to effectively manage the people risks, and make a real difference to care and business outcomes? The model healthcare employer must have in place a number of key mechanisms (see box overleaf).

Action along these lines will help ensure that health organisations are more attractive places to work, encouraging recruitment, retention and morale. It will also contribute to the ability to move forward, taking account of lessons from the past, and to greater organisational success for the future.

Key human resource strategies to underpin risk management

- sound recruitment and selection procedures, including pre-employment checks, training in equality and interview skills and good induction

- systems for learning from errors, including blame culture eradication, appraisal and retraining, and for keeping up to date with legislation and other developments

- strategies for adequate resourcing, including employee attraction and retention, a balanced skill mix and continuous monitoring of job content and workload through performance review

- effective performance based on high-quality teams, high-quality leadership and sound supervision

- action to improve morale by good communications and staff involvement

- a comprehensive range of human resource policies, including those to tackle sickness absence and discrimination

---

References

See also KEY REFERENCES, piii

1. Department of Health (2001) *Investment and reform for NHS Staff – taking forward the NHS Plan,* DoH, Leeds.

2. The Allitt Inquiry (1994) *The Allitt Inquiry, Independent inquiry relating to deaths and injuries on the children's ward at Grantham and Kesteven General Hospital during the period February to April 1991,* HMSO, London.

3. Bullock, R (1997) *Report of the independent inquiry into the major employment and ethical issues arising from the events leading to the trial of Amanda Jenkinson,* North Nottinghamshire Health Authority, Nottingham.

4. Commission for Health Improvement (2001) *Employing locum consultants – matters arising from the employment of Dr Elwood,* CHI, London. (*www.chi.nhs.uk*)

5. *Code of Practice in HCHS Locum Doctor Appointment and Employment,* NHS Executive, August 1997.

6. HSG (92) 31 Employment of medical and dental staff, NHS Management Executive, July 1992.

7. Redfern, M (2001) *The report of The Royal Liverpool Children's Inquiry,* HMSO, London. (*www.rlcinquiry.org.uk*)

8. Office of the Commissioner for Public Appointments (2001) *OCPA Code of*

practice for ministerial appointments to public bodies, OCPA, London. (*www.ocpa.gov.uk*)

9. Department of Health (2001) *Assuring the quality of medical practice,* HMSO, London.

10. Health Service Circular 2000/019, *Appointment procedures for hospital and community medical and dental staff*

11. Penna Sanders & Sidney (1998) *Surviving the honeymoon: research report,* Penna Sanders & Sidney, London.

12. Department of Health (1999) *Supporting doctors, protecting patients,* HMSO, London.

13. Deeks, E (2001) 'Solitary lessons in how to manage your weaknesses', *People Management,* 17 May.

14. *Proposals for a new duty to investigate, accidents, dangerous occurrences and diseases,* HSE consultative document (CD 169), May 2001.

15. Improving Working Lives Standard, DoH, September 2001.

16. Department of Health (2001) *Code of practice for NHS employers involved in the international recruitment of healthcare professionals,* DoH, London.

17. Buchan, J (2000) *Determining skill mix in the health workforce: guidelines for managers and health professionals (discussion paper 3),* World Health Organisation, Geneva.

18. *Employee absence: a survey of management policy and practice,* CIPD, June 2001.

Further information

Roberts, G (1997) *Recruitment and selection, a competency approach,* Chartered Institute for Personnel and Development, London.

Burford, B, Bullas, S, Collier, B (2000) *Positively diverse report 2000,* NHS Executive, Leeds.

Department of Trade and Industry (1999) *Regulation of the private recruitment Industry, a consultation document,* DTI, London.

Audit Commission (1999) *Brief encounters: getting the best from temporary nursing staff,* Audit Commission, London.

Penna Sanders & Sidney (1998) *Surviving the honeymoon: research report,* Penna Sanders & Sidney, London.

Johnson, R (2001) 'On Message – internal communications', *People management,* 30 August.

Labour Research Department (2001) *Law at work,* London.

Glossary

Adverse healthcare event, an untoward incident associated with healthcare delivery. An event or omission arising during clinical care and causing physical or psychological injury to a patient.

Business continuity management, the process by which arrangements are made to ensure service delivery following major disruption to normal business activity

Clinical governance, the application of the principles of corporate governance to clinical risk, with the overall aim of enhancing the quality of patient care delivery

Clinical risk, risk specifically associated with clinical practice or patient care delivery

Clinical risk management, a systematic process where clinical risk is identified and measures introduced to reduce risk with the overall aim of improving patient care

Continuous professional development, the development of personal programmes of training and development for professional staff, including clinicians and healthcare staff, to ensure their professional practice remains up to date

Controls assurance, the approach to corporate governance developed within the NHS. A verification process to test that NHS organisations are effectively managing risk.

Corporate governance, a holistic approach to developing systems of internal control within an organisation and to the verification of the effectiveness of these systems

Credentialling, the verification during recruitment of an individual's identity, qualifications and experience in order to ensure the quality of healthcare provision

Crisis management, the strategic response in the immediate aftermath of a major incident

Drug error, a mistake in administration of patient medication

Error, a mistake either intended or unintended that leads to an adverse outcome. Errors can be both active and have immediate effect or latent where the consequences become apparent after a period of time.

Hazard, the potential to cause harm

Hazard identification, the process by which hazards are determined or spotted

Human factors, environmental, organisational and job factors, and human and individual characteristics which influence behaviour at work in a way that can affect risk

Incident, undesired circumstances which may or may not cause harm

Near-miss, an accident with the potential to cause harm or damage

Risk, the probability or chance that harm will arise

Risk assessment, the systematic identification of the causes of harm and additional measures necessary to remove or reduce risk

Risk management, the systematic identification, evaluation and treatment of risk. A continuous process with the aim of reducing risk to organisations and individuals alike.

Root cause, the immediate underlying cause of an incident or accident that can be readily identified and is within the ability of managers and staff to fix

Service continuity management, a term interchangeable with business continuity management, most usually used in service organisations

Service continuity plans, the identification of the systematic steps to be planned and followed in order to ensure continuity of service provision

Service recovery, a term interchangeable with business recovery, involving the arrangements to be put in place to ensure continuity of service provision following major disruption

Skill mix, the blend of skills needed amongst a team of staff to ensure effective healthcare delivery

Supply chain, the interdependent relationship between organisations supplying goods and services

Index of Acts and Regulations

General Index